THE
Red Wine Diet

Rosemary Conley

ARROW

Published in the United Kingdom in 2000
by Arrow Books

1 3 5 7 9 10 8 6 4 2

First published in the United Kingdom in 2000 by Arrow

Arrow Books
The Random House Group Limited
20 Vauxhall Bridge Road, London SW1V 2SA

Random House, Australia (Pty) Limited
20 Afred Street, Milsons Point, Sydney,
New South Wales 2061, Australia

Random House New Zealand Limited
18 Poland Road, Glenfield, Auckland 10, New Zealand

Random House (Pty) Limited
Endulini, 5a Jubilee Road, Parktown 2193, South Africa

The Random House Group Limited Reg. No. 954009
www.randomhouse.co.uk

A CIP catalogue record for this book is available
from the British Library

Papers used by Random House are natural, recyclable products
made from wood grown in sustainable forests. The manufacturing
processes conform to the environmental regulations of the country
of origin

Printed and bound in Denmark by
Nørhaven A/S, Viborg

ISBN 0 09 940609 8

Design/make up by Roger Walker
Illustrations by Leslie Dean

Contents

Acknowledgements

I extend my most grateful thanks to the many people without whom this book would not have been possible.

Firstly to my assistant, Melody Patterson, for organising the Trial Diet and gathering together the material I needed for typing my manuscript; to my PA, Louise Jones, for helping to compile the results of the trial; to chef Dean Simpole-Clarke for contributing many of the recipes; and to Mary Morris, my fitness consultant, for her most valuable contribution to the exercise section.

Further thanks must go to Dr Kevin Sykes of University College, Chester, for his help, encouragement and contribution; and special thanks to Dr Susan Jebb of the MRC Human Nutrition and Research Centre in Cambridge for checking that the nutrition information is consistent with the latest scientific evidence.

Special thanks also must go to my long-suffering editor, Jan Bowmer, for yet again transforming one of my manuscripts into a readable book. Thank you also to art director Dennis Barker and designer Roger Walker.

Last, but by no means least, a big thank you to all the men who participated in my Trial Diet. Their encouraging remarks, dedication to the cause and their ultimate success motivated me to write this book. Thank you all.

Foreword

The 1997 Health Survey for England showed that more than six out of 10 men are overweight and at increased risk of a whole range of serious diseases such as heart attack and diabetes. Excess weight is also associated with a number of other conditions that may not be life-threatening but which do decrease the quality of every-day life. These range from joint problems that limit mobility, to snoring, which leads to domestic disputes and sleepless nights!

It follows that tackling the problem is not just about losing weight but also about improving health. This book contains valuable information to help you become slimmer and fitter. Rosemary Conley has adapted her successful diet and fitness philosophy for women to produce a programme for men. The low-fat eating plan in this book includes plenty of complex car-bohydrates to maintain bulk in the diet and keep hunger at bay and closely follows current nutritional guidelines. This is not a short-term diet but a long-term eating plan to help you achieve and maintain a healthy weight.

Susan A. Jebb, PhD, SRD
MRC Human Nutrition Research Centre, Cambridge

1

How to Lose Weight without Starving

Please tick the boxes alongside the statements that apply to you:

1 I adore food ☐
2 I have a large appetite ☐
3 I hate feeling hungry ☐
4 I don't want to diet ☐
5 I don't want to give up alcohol ☐
6 I don't want to go jogging ☐
7 I do want to lose some weight ☐
8 I would like to be healthier ☐
9 I would like to be fitter ☐

If you have ticked most of these boxes, this book is for you.

Personally, I would have ticked all the boxes! I love my food and I know what it is like to be overweight and unhappy with your figure. In 1986, however, I discovered the enormous benefits of 'eating low fat'. I was advised to follow a low-fat diet in order to avoid surgery for gallstones. Not only did my health improve dramatically, but the unexpected additional benefit was that I also lost loads of inches from my previously outsized hips and thighs, an area I had been trying to slim down for 20 years! Simply by following a very low-fat diet, I transformed my shape.

Perhaps the most remarkable thing was that, although I lost only 6lb, I looked as if I had lost a stone! The change in my figure was quite astonishing. When the ladies who attended my slimming and exercise classes noticed this transformation they pleaded with me to share my secret. I designed a diet for them; they changed shape, just as I had; and I knew I'd hit on something special.

I then conducted some trials, enrolling volunteer dieters through local radio in my hometown of Leicester and in nearby Nottingham. Women flocked to try this 'miracle' diet and husbands joined in. 'Well, if you're doing it, I might as well lose a few pounds too,' was a typical response from many male partners.

After following the diet for eight weeks, my trial dieters completed a questionnaire. The results were incredible. Everybody lost weight, but, again, it was the inch loss that was astounding. The women all *looked* so much slimmer. Even the men who followed the diet in a half-hearted kind of a way lost weight and inches. It was truly the start of a dietary revolution.

Many women wrote additional comments on the questionnaire. 'My husband says I now have the figure I had when I married him 25 years ago,' wrote one woman gleefully. Another wrote: 'My husband followed the diet with me. I am pleased to report that he has regained his boyish figure after 30 years! I'm thrilled!' But perhaps the comment that made the deepest impression on me was that from a lady who wrote: 'I can't stop looking in the mirror.' She was 79 years old! You can imagine my excitement at the results.

I then wrote my *Hip and Thigh Diet*, which was first published in 1988, and its sequel, *Rosemary Conley's Complete Hip and Thigh Diet*, a year later. Between them, these two books have sold almost 2.5 million copies, which must say something of their effectiveness. Eating a low-fat diet has the effect of quickly and healthily streamlining the body.

In recent years scientists have conducted many trials on the role of fat in the diet and how easily the body stores it. The results are conclusive and the medical profession is now united in recommending low-fat eating as a safe and effective way of losing weight. Obesity has a detrimental effect on our health and we are given every encouragement to lose our excess weight and make some modifications to our regular eating patterns as well as increase our activity levels. Becoming more active helps control body weight, but it also has independent effects on fitness and wellbeing. Anyone who exercises regularly will become leaner and fitter, even if their weight remains unaltered.

We live in an age when food has never been so plentiful in the western world. Prolific advertising and all too easily available high-fat snack foods on every corner and at every petrol station are tempting us to snack or feast. But, sadly, a high-fat diet does more than make us fat; it contributes to high cholesterol levels and furring up of the arteries. And if we are overweight we are more likely to suffer medical conditions such as high blood pressure, diabetes and heart disease.

The good news is that I don't advocate making drastic changes to your eating patterns, only that you make some modifications and also undertake moderate amounts of activity. I want to encourage you to eat well and enjoy life. I am not for a moment suggesting that you have to live on lettuce leaves and cottage cheese or start training for the London Marathon! I couldn't do that and I don't expect you to!

At the beginning of this chapter I asked you to answer some questions. Now I would like you to consider whether you are a 'live to eat' type of person or whether you are someone who just 'eats to live'. I am definitely the former, as food plays a very important part in my life. I look forward to each meal and enjoy every mouthful. I rarely leave anything on my plate, and if there is a particular dish I adore, I can always find a space for a second helping.

On the other hand, I know many people who are quite indifferent towards food. They eat only because their stomach tells them they must, they often leave a couple of mouthfuls at the side of the plate because they have had sufficient, and they often decline the dessert. These people usually stay slim quite naturally and are looked upon by many as being incredibly lucky that they don't have to struggle with their weight. Under closer scrutiny, it is plain to see why they remain slim. It is because they simply eat less than the 'live to eat' brigade. But some men seem to eat loads of food and yet stay thin. Is their metabolic rate so much faster than the norm that they just burn up the calories?

These theories have been put to the test in numerous studies at the MRC Dunn Nutrition Centre in Cambridge using a whole-body calorimeter. A whole-body calorimeter is a sealed unit rather like a small bed-sitting room with wash basin, TV, bed, exercise bike, and so on. Here the oxygen and carbon dioxide intake and expenditure can be accurately monitored and body energy expenditure calculated. Volunteers are fed regularly through a two-way hatch and their waste matter is passed out through the hatch in appropriate containers!

One study by Erik Diaz, which was published in the American Journal of Clinical Nutrition in 1992, took two groups of men – one lean and one overweight. All the men were overfed in excess of 50 per cent of their energy needs, by increasing the total amount of food in their diet, and they all gained weight at the same rate. There are two important points to note. The first is that the lean men who had claimed they 'could eat like a horse and never gain weight', gained weight at the same rate as those who said 'I only look at a meat pie and gain weight'. Lean people do not have any special mechanism that allows them to burn off excess calories without getting fat. Secondly, the study shows that, although some people believe they are eating as much as they like, they are in fact eating exactly the correct amount to meet their energy requirements. The interesting question arising from this study is, what is the mechanism that allows some people to subconsciously eat exactly the right amount for their energy needs, when others (probably the majority) always tend to eat a little (or a lot) more than appropriate?

Another study by James Stubbs, which was published in the American Journal of Clinical Nutrition in 1995, involved six lean men. They were given diets containing different proportions of fat on three occasions for a week each time. The study was carried out twice. The first time, the volunteers were confined in a whole-body calorimeter. The second time, the study was carried out under normal living conditions.

On each occasion the proportion of fat in the men's diet was secretly changed from low (20 per cent of the total calories) to medium (40 per cent of the total calories) and high (60 per cent of the total calories). The volunteers were allowed to eat whenever they wanted and as much or as little as they wished. On the low-fat diet they lost weight each time, despite eating as much as they wished. On the medium-fat diet, while the men were in the calorimeter, they gained a little weight, but outside the calorimeter their weight remained roughly constant (presumably because, when confined to a calorimeter, the men were less active and, consequently, burned off less energy). On the high-fat diet the men gained weight on both occasions (both inside and outside the calorimeter). In fact, the weight (bulk) of food they consumed was similar on each occasion, but because the meals that were high in fat were more energy dense than the low- or medium-fat meals (i.e. they contained more calories per gram because of the higher fat content), the men consumed more calories on the high-fat diet and therefore gained weight.

Scientists working with animals have also observed the detrimental effects of a high-fat diet. In studies where rats were fed an unlimited diet of standard rat pellets for a period of time, the rats always maintained a healthy weight (even though more pellets were always available). At certain times their food supply was reduced and the rats lost weight, as you would expect. As soon as the normal food supply was resumed the rats tucked in, eating as much as they liked, and each rat's weight increased, but only to its previous level, until the food was removed again for another period of 'dieting'. The experiment was repeated three times. During each of the three 'dieting' periods, the weight of the rats dropped, and as soon as they returned to normal eating their weight rose again to exactly the same level as before. Their weight did not increase beyond that norm. But when the scientists introduced high-fat food such as cheese and chocolate chip cookies, the rats found them so delicious they just kept eating them, and because they continued to eat the cookies, their weight just went up and up.

The lesson to learn is that if we are given uninspiring food we will probably not eat much of it because we'll get bored. Our built-in appestat, located in the brain, determines when we have had sufficient food. But if we taste something that is really scrumptious, we override our natural appestat and just eat more of the delicious food. If we do this regularly our weight will obviously increase dramatically, just as the rats' weight did.

It would be simple to say that the answer to weight loss is to put ourselves on a boring diet and the weight will automatically come off. However, for many of us, that is simply not practical. We lead varied lives where we might eat a sandwich in the office one day and be wined and dined for lunch the next. Our daily pattern of eating is a potential minefield and we need to learn how we can walk through it in order to minimise the danger yet still feel that we are satisfied both physically and psychologically. We don't want to feel hungry, we don't want rabbit food, and we don't want to feel deprived.

That is why I have included three separate diet plans in this book. The first, the No Diet Diet, is for those men who just wouldn't stick to a diet but need some overall guidance on what to eat. The second, the Bachelor's Diet, is for men who live on their own, who do not have a great deal of time to spend on cooking and find heating up a ready-made meal in the microwave a great option. The third, the Gourmet Diet, is for those who enjoy cooking and have time to go shopping for the ingredients or who have a partner who can do this for them. Although I have designed these diets with men in mind, women can certainly follow any of them by reducing the portion sizes by 25 per cent.

The next obvious question is why have I called this book the Red Wine Diet? Well, it's because red wine is actually good for us. Red wine has been proven to have some real benefits to health, from helping to stave off heart attacks and strokes to giving protection against some cancers. In addition red wine is high in antioxidants, which very effectively zap the potentially cancer-giving free radicals that occur naturally in the body. The substance which is responsible for the colour of red grape skins is packed full of antioxidants. These transfer to the wine and suddenly your glass of wine becomes a health drink! Good news all round. That is why you are allowed three glasses of red wine a day (two for women) when following any of the three diet plans in this book, although if you prefer, you can substitute three units of any other alcohol (two units for women).

Before I outline the diets themselves I'd like to explain some simple principles on how they work – if you are thinking of skipping this bit, please don't! If you understand the effects of fat and calories on the body, you are more likely to make some changes to your lifestyle.

Calories, metabolism, and all that stuff!

A calorie is a unit of energy and is used to measure the energy value of food. Its full title is 'kilocalorie' (kcal), which is why nutrition panels on food packaging indicate the number of 'kcal'. In everyday language, though, we simply refer to it as a calorie.

Are all calories equal?

It was by accident that I discovered that low-fat eating leads to a leaner body. Fortunately, scientists are now able to illustrate how the body uses carbohydrate calories and burns them off rather than storing them, while the body is extremely efficient at storing fat.

At one time it was thought that, provided you ate fewer calories than your body burned up each day, you would lose weight and that it didn't matter what made up those calories – it could be chocolate or chips, as long as you didn't exceed your calorie allowance. It is certainly true that if we eat fewer calories than our body burns up each day we will lose weight. BUT – and it is a big but – this old way of thinking did not take into account the fact that 'weight loss' on the scales is not representative of 'fat loss' from the body. We can lose weight through a reduction in bodily fluids, muscle tissue and fat, but fat is much less useful to us than muscle. Interestingly, a kilogram of fat contains 9,000 calories, while a kilogram of muscle has about 1,000 calories.

On a weight-loss plan there are three main reasons why we want to lose body fat. Firstly, we don't need so much of it. Secondly, compared with muscle, it uses fewer calories to sustain it and, thirdly, it is ugly and unhealthy. On the other hand, lean muscle tissue is something to be treasured; it demands lots of calories to sustain it – in fact, weight for weight, muscle burns three times as many calories as those burned by fat. Muscle is hungry tissue that keeps our metabolic rate buoyant and uses energy even when we are not exercising. During exercise, the energy expenditure of muscle increases dramatically, but there is very little change in the energy expenditure of fat. Muscle burns 13 calories per kilogram of body weight per day, while fat burns just 4.5 calories per kilogram.

Fat is very easily stored by the body for emergencies. In its evolutionary process, the body was designed to store fat to keep energy supplies ready for times of famine. Sounds far-fetched? Well here is further proof.

In 1996 I made a series of films for ITV's *This Morning* programme. I went along with a film crew to the MRC Dunn Nutrition Centre in Cambridge where Dr Andrew Prentice, who at that time was Head of the Energy Metabolism Research Group, showed us an experiment. A volunteer was given a high-carbohydrate meal – a plate of pasta. After the volunteer had eaten the meal, a plastic hood with a breathing tube connected to a computer (called a metabolic hood) was placed over his head. As he continued to breathe quite normally the computer registered an increase in energy expenditure, signifying that the carbohydrate was being burned off.

A similar test was run on another volunteer. This time the volunteer was given a bar of chocolate that was high in fat but which contained the same number of calories as the plate of pasta. Again the metabolic hood was placed over the volunteer's head, but the machine did not show any change in energy expenditure! In other words, the body had absorbed all the fat from the chocolate without burning any extra calories.

The pitfalls of crash dieting

Most people who decide to shed a few pounds want to do it fast! There is an understandable temptation to eat fewer and fewer calories in the belief that the less you eat the more weight you lose. There are three main problems with this theory. Firstly, eating too little stretches your willpower to its limits, leaves you feeling very hungry and deprived and always – yes, always – ends in disaster when the inevitable eating binge takes over. A sense of failure, desperation and disappointment follow and your good intentions are replaced by a feeling of resignation that you are meant to be fat!

The second problem is that the body doesn't like being starved and automatically changes down a gear towards self-preservation. The body becomes as efficient as possible and tries not to waste a single calorie.

In fact, on the most severe diets, your metabolic rate can actually decrease by up to 20 per cent.

There is yet another problem. Since there isn't enough energy in your food, your body takes the energy it needs from its reserves. Normally, this would come from its fat stores, but during rapid weight loss brought about by crash dieting, the energy comes from the muscles. Yes, you lose weight on the scales – possibly lots of it – but it is weight from the wrong places. The worst news of all is that the less muscle you have, the lower your metabolic rate. Crash dieting – eating fewer than 800 calories a day for a woman and 1,200 calories for a man – is bad news on all sides. It is counterproductive, it doesn't re-educate your eating habits, and because you don't actually lose much body fat, it doesn't work in the long term. Anyway, why crash diet when you can lose weight much more efficiently by eating more?

How many calories can I eat and still lose weight?

The average man burns around 1,700–2,000 calories a day just by being alive – even if he stays in bed all day. We call this the basal metabolic rate (BMR). The average BMR for women is around 1,400 calories a day. As soon as you get out of bed and go about your daily work, you burn even more. The more active you are, the more calories you burn. The total number of calories you burn each day is referred to as your total energy expenditure. It includes calories burned both at rest and during physical activity.

Another interesting fact is that the heavier you are, the more calories your body needs, rather like a large car uses more fuel than a small one. On pages 20–25 you will find tables giving you an approximate calculation of your basic daily calorie requirements, depending on your weight and age. Use these to calculate your basal (resting) metabolic rate. There is also a column indicating your likely calorie expenditure in a typical day. Just decide whether you are sedentary, active or very active. Obviously the more active you are, the more calories you will spend. I have included charts for women too.

Losing weight is a simple matter of physics. Your body needs a certain number of calories to keep you alive and give you the energy to live your daily life. If you eat more calories than your body uses, you will gain weight, and if you eat fewer calories than your body uses, you will lose weight. If you eat an equal number of calories to those you use, your body weight will remain constant.

Sometimes your weight will remain constant when you think you should be losing it. When this happens, then I'm afraid you are probably deceiving yourself. You are simply likely to be eating more calories than you think you are and you are not being active enough!

How can I maximise my weight loss?

You can lose body fat effectively by eating sufficient low-fat calories to make your body believe that it is not dieting and you can burn extra calories by doing more activity. The most efficient way to lose body fat, therefore, is to eat a low-fat diet of around 2,000 calories a day for men (1,400 calories for women) and combine this with 30 minutes of physical activity, at a level that makes you slightly breathless, three to five times a week.

In all my diets, I adopt two key criteria. One is that I stipulate a calorie allowance that is equal to the basal metabolic rate of the average man or woman (the number of calories your body would burn up if you stayed in bed all day) and I also select ingredients that usually contain a maximum of 4 per cent fat – 4g fat per 100g food. On this basis, my dieters have plenty of food to eat, the diet is naturally low in fat, but the body receives sufficient nutrition for health and to satisfy its basic needs. The extra energy that is expended through your daily activities and any other exercise you take will be drawn from your fat stores. If you eat low fat, then your fat stores will not be replenished through the food that you eat.

As a rough guide, this is how I allocate the daily calories in a typical diet.

	Men	Women
300ml (½ pint) of skimmed or semi-skimmed milk (450ml/¾ pint for women)	150 kcal	225 kcal
3 units of alcohol (2 for women)	300 kcal	200 kcal
Breakfast	300 kcal	225 kcal
Lunch	450 kcal	300 kcal
Dinner (including dessert)	600 kcal	450 kcal
Treats (none for women)	200 kcal	Nil
TOTAL	2000 kcal	1400 kcal

The calories can be moved around and the alcoholic drinks are optional. However, if you do not take your alcoholic drinks I do not recommend that you replace those calories with additional food. Alcohol is utilised by the body quite differently from food. The body regards alcohol as a poison and therefore works hard to get rid of it as quickly as possible. It will process and dispose of alcohol in preference to burning carbohydrates, proteins or fats. However, it would be wrong to think that calories from alcohol don't count, because they definitely do (more about this later).

There is no need to be too regimental about your daily calorie intake. If one day you take in 1,600 calories and on another day 1,800 calories, it really doesn't matter. Just try and average it over the week. To lose just over 1kg (2lb) a week the average man needs to eat 7,700 fewer calories per week than his body spends. This is how it works. See it as a balance sheet.

ENERGY OUTGOINGS PER DAY FOR MEN
based on an 11½ stone man

	OUTGOINGS (kcal)		INCOME (kcal)
Energy spent in being alive (basal metabolic rate)	1,700	Food consumed	1,700
Energy spent in going about your everyday tasks	1,200	Alcohol allowance	300
Exercise 3–5 times a week plus additional physical activity (average per day)	200		
Total	3,100	Total	2,000
		Shortfall of income (food etc.) over expenditure (calories burned) = potential weight loss from body	1,100
TOTAL ENERGY SPENT	3,100		3,100

An energy deficit of 1,100 calories a day represents a deficit of 7,700 calories a week and a weight loss of 1kg (2lb), which on a low-fat diet will mostly be body fat.

Can I lose weight by dieting alone?

By following a diet of 2,000 calories a day, a man will go into debt by only approximately 6,100 calories a week. To reach a target of 1kg (2lb) fat loss per week he would need to spend another 1,400 calories during the course of the week. This is where exercise comes in.

The key to exercise is to find a form of activity that you enjoy. If you exercise on a regular basis you will definitely lose weight faster *and* you will lose more fat from your body. You will look and feel so good that you will be encouraged to continue on your healthy campaign. So, get into the habit of doing some exercise on a regular basis, but don't feel that you have to train for the Olympics! Exercise is recommended on only three to five days a week, as the body needs two rest days to restock its energy stores, rather like recharging a battery. Ideally, exercise three days on and one day off. The exercise programme in Chapter 6 of this book is based on exercising five times a week and shows you how to strike a balance between aerobic exercise and muscle strengthening exercise.

Now here's some more good news. If you are very overweight you will actually burn more calories than your slim friend for the same amount of activity, because it requires more energy to move a bigger body. This means you won't have to work so hard to achieve the same results, so don't exhaust yourself. Remember that any activity is better than none, and the one you enjoy doing is the very best one for you because you are more likely to keep on doing it.

I think I have a slow metabolism. Is that possible?

Our metabolic rate is the rate at which we burn our food, rather like the number of miles per gallon a car can do. Like a car, the bigger the body, the more fuel it uses. Our bodies use a lot of energy just to tick over – to keep the heart beating, bones and tissue renewing, food processing, and so on. The approximate number of calories used by the body for this process is between 1,700 and 2,000 for men, depending on their size. The more muscle a man has, the higher his metabolic rate.

Many people put their overweight problem down to a slow metabolic rate, but, in honesty, in 99·9 per cent of the cases, the reason people are overweight is simply that they eat too much and do too little!

At the MRC Dunn Nutrition Centre in Cambridge many studies and clinical tests have been undertaken on metabolism and weight loss. Firstly, it was concluded that it is extraordinarily rare for anyone to have a lower than average metabolism. Secondly, in tests where both overweight and slim people were asked to keep daily diet diaries the results were very interesting. Slim people accurately recorded what they ate, while the overweight volunteers, on average, underestimated how much they ate by a third!

Although many overweight people think they have a slow metabolic rate, in fact the reverse is true. If you have a big, heavy body, you will burn more calories than someone who is smaller and lighter. The good news is that you can lose weight without starving. You can maintain your metabolic rate so that you can still eat plenty of food when you are slim, and feel fit and healthy into the bargain.

Interesting information has now come to light regarding the maintenance of our metabolic rate after we have lost weight. Naturally, as our body weight reduces our energy requirement also reduces, because there is less of us to move around. The good news is that we can counter this by taking regular exercise. It has been proved that people who exercise while they diet do not reduce their metabolic rate, providing the diet they follow offers sufficient calories (like the diet plans in this book). However, anyone who diets without taking exercise will suffer a reduction in their metabolic rate, and those who crash diet will find that reduction significantly greater. Exercise also has many additional benefits to weight maintenance, which I will explain more fully in Chapter 6.

Overweight people blame many things for their size and here are the ten most common excuses I have heard in my 25 or so years in the business.

1 I have a slow metabolism.
2 I can't exercise because . . . .
3 I am taking medication for . . . .
4 It's my glands.
5 I don't have time to diet.
6 I hardly eat anything anyway.
7 It's my job – I work irregular hours.
8 It's not fat, it's muscle.
9 It's in my genes.
10 I have tried many diets and diets don't work for me.

I believe the problem of excess weight arises not from a slow metabolism or lack of exercise; it comes from our attitude to food. If we really love food – any food – then the chances are that we will have a weight problem, because it takes willpower to stop eating when we are enjoying ourselves. Some people keep on eating when they don't need to; some people keep on spending money even when they can't afford to; others can't stop drinking when they have had more than enough. Addiction? Possibly. We have to eat food to stay alive, but we have to learn to control our urges.

Motivation: the key to success

Why is it that the more you want to lose weight and the more you try, the more you seem to struggle, often with the result that your weight increases rather than decreases? This often occurs simply because we become more conscious of the food that we are eating and the restraints that a weight-loss programme inflicts upon us. The key is to find a reason for losing your excess weight, setting a goal and looking at the benefits – real benefits – of achieving that goal.

The decision to go on a diet and lose weight is usually triggered by something specific, such as seeing a photograph of yourself, finding that a pair of trousers you haven't worn for a few months just won't zip up, you get 'stuck' in something – a seat, a turnstile, whatever – or you see yourself on video. Or it could be something physical where you suddenly have to run to help rescue somebody, chase someone, or catch up with a

Daily energy (kilocalorie) requirements of men aged 18–29 years

Body weight (stones)	BMR	Total energy requirement (kcal per day)		
		Sedentary	Active	Very Active
8	1456	2180	2480	2770
8.5	1509	2260	2570	2870
9	1557	2340	2650	2960
9.5	1606	2410	2730	3050
10	1652	2480	2810	3140
10.5	1701	2550	2890	3230
11	1749	2620	2970	3320
11.5	1797	2700	3060	3410
12	1846	2770	3140	3510
12.5	1892	2840	3220	3600
13	1940	2910	3300	3690
13.5	1990	2980	3380	3780
14	2037	3060	3460	3870
14.5	2086	3130	3550	3960
15	2134	3200	3630	4050
15.5	2180	3270	3710	4140
16	2220	3330	3770	4220
16.5	2278	3420	3870	4330
17	2330	3490	3950	4420
17.5	2365	3548	4020	4494
18	2410	3615	4097	4579
18.5	2460	3690	4182	4674
19	2510	3765	4267	4769
19.5	2555	3832	4344	4854
20	2605	3908	4428	4950

Daily energy (kilocalorie) requirements of men aged 30–59 years

Body weight (stones)	BMR	Total energy requirement (kcal per day)		
		Sedentary	Active	Very Active
8	1458	2190	2480	2770
8.5	1495	2240	2540	2840
9	1532	2300	2600	2910
9.5	1569	2350	2670	2980
10	1604	2410	2730	3050
10.5	1641	2460	2790	3120
11	1678	2520	2850	3190
11.5	1715	2570	2920	3260
12	1752	2630	2980	3330
12.5	1787	2680	3040	3400
13	1824	2740	3100	3470
13.5	1861	2790	3160	3540
14	1898	2850	3230	3640
14.5	1934	2900	3290	3680
15	1970	2960	3350	3750
15.5	2007	3010	3410	3810
16	2037	3060	3460	3870
16.5	2080	3120	3540	3950
17	2117	3180	3600	4020
17.5	2150	3225	3655	4085
18	2184	3276	3713	4150
18.5	2220	3330	3774	4218
19	2260	3390	3842	4294
19.5	2295	3442	3902	4360
20	2330	3495	3961	4427

Daily energy (kilocalorie) requirements of men aged 60 years and over

Body weight (stones)	BMR	Total energy requirement (kcal per day)		
		Sedentary	Active	Very Active
8	1182	1773	2009	2246
8.5	1220	1830	2074	2318
9	1256	1884	2135	2386
9.5	1294	1941	2200	2459
10	1331	1996	2263	2529
10.5	1368	2052	2326	2599
11	1406	2109	2390	2671
11.5	1443	2164	2453	2742
12	1480	2220	2516	2812
12.5	1517	2276	2579	2882
13	1555	2332	2644	2954
13.5	1591	2386	2705	3023
14	1629	2444	2769	3095
14.5	1666	2499	2832	3165
15	1704	2556	2897	3238
15.5	1740	2610	2958	3306
16	1777	2666	3021	3376
16.5	1815	2722	3086	3448
17	1852	2778	3148	3519
17.5	1888	2832	3210	3587
18	1926	2889	3274	3659
18.5	1964	2946	3339	3732
19	2000	3000	3400	3800
19.5	2038	3057	3465	3872
20	2075	3112	3528	3942

Daily energy (kilocalorie) requirements of women aged 18–29 years

Body weight (stones)	BMR	Total energy requirement (kcal per day) Sedentary	Active	Very Active
7	1146	1720	1950	2180
7.5	1193	1790	2030	2270
8	1240	1860	2110	2360
8.5	1288	1930	2190	2450
9	1335	2000	2270	2540
9.5	1382	2070	2350	2630
10	1428	2140	2430	2710
10.5	1476	2210	2510	2800
11	1523	2280	2590	2890
11.5	1570	2360	2670	2980
12	1618	2430	2750	3070
12.5	1664	2500	2830	3160
13	1711	2570	2830	3250
13.5	1758	2640	2990	3340
14	1806	2710	3070	3430
14.5	1853	2780	3150	3520
15	1900	2850	3230	3610
15.5	1945	2918	3306	3696
16	1992	2988	3386	3785
16.5	2040	3060	3468	3876
17	2087	3130	3548	3965
17.5	2133	3200	3628	4053
18	2180	3270	3706	4142
18.5	2228	3342	3788	4233
19	2274	3411	3866	4321
19.5	2320	3480	3944	4408
20	2370	3555	4029	4503

Daily energy (kilocalorie) requirements of women aged 30–59 years

Body weight		Total energy requirement (kcal per day)		
(stones)	BMR	Sedentary	Active	Very Active
7	1215	1820	2070	2310
7.5	1242	1860	2110	2360
8	1268	1900	2160	2410
8.5	1295	1940	2200	2460
9	1323	1980	2250	2510
9.5	1348	2020	2290	2560
10	1374	2060	2340	2610
10.5	1400	2100	2380	2660
11	1427	2140	2430	2710
11.5	1454	2180	2470	2760
12	1480	2220	2520	2810
12.5	1505	2260	2560	2860
13	1532	2300	2600	2910
13.5	1559	2340	2650	2960
14	1586	2380	2700	3010
14.5	1612	2420	2740	3060
15	1639	2460	2790	3110
15.5	1645	2468	2796	3126
16	1671	2506	2841	3175
16.5	1700	2550	2890	3230
17	1723	2584	2929	3274
17.5	1750	2625	2975	3325
18	1774	2661	3016	3371
18.5	1800	2700	3060	3420
19	1825	2738	3102	3468
19.5	1852	2778	3148	3519
20	1880	2820	3196	3572

Daily energy (kilocalorie) requirements of women aged 60 years and over

Body weight (stones)	BMR	Total energy requirement (kcal per day)		
		Sedentary	Active	Very Active
7	998	1500	1700	1900
7.5	1028	1542	1750	1950
8	1057	1590	1800	2010
8.5	1087	1630	1850	2070
9	1116	1670	1900	2120
9.5	1146	1720	1950	2180
10	1174	1760	2000	2230
10.5	1204	1810	2050	2290
11	1233	1850	2100	2340
11.5	1263	1890	2150	2400
12	1292	1940	2200	2450
12.5	1320	1980	2240	2510
13	1350	2030	2300	2570
13.5	1380	2070	2350	2620
14	1409	2110	2400	2680
14.5	1439	2160	2450	2730
15	1469	2200	2500	2790
15.5	1552	2328	2638	2949
16	1581	2372	2688	3004
16.5	1610	2415	2737	3059
17	1639	2458	2786	3114
17.5	1667	2500	2834	3167
18	1697	2546	2885	3224
18.5	1726	2589	2934	3279
19	1754	2631	2982	3333
19.5	1783	2674	3031	3388
20	1810	2715	3077	3439

friend, and you realise that you can't get your breath and your fitness has left you. Another motivating factor could be your GP or the doctor who examined you for that recent medical check-up and told you fairly and squarely that if you didn't lose weight and get fitter you might not live as long as you thought you would. It is usually something that gives you a real shock which makes you take action. That is the point when you actually face up to the problem and say 'enough is enough' and decide to do something about it. Nobody can make the decision for you – you have to make it yourself. To succeed in losing weight, you have to want to do it badly enough.

At the time you may think this is only happening to you. Well, it has probably happened to most readers of this book. So you are not alone and you are definitely not a hopeless case. I have helped hundreds of thousands of women to lose weight very successfully over the last few years, and if my diets can work for them, there is absolutely no reason why they shouldn't work for you too!

To make a fresh start on *your* diet and fitness campaign you need to make some changes in your life. Here are some suggestions that might help.

★ Recognise the times when you are tempted to indulge in those high-fat treats that you know have contributed to your weight problem. If you always buy your daily newspaper from a shop that sells chocolate and you usually end up buying a bar, shop somewhere else. Make a break and stop buying that KitKat!

★ Don't be tempted to buy too many low-fat or fat-free snacks. They may be low in fat but they are still high in calories. If they are in the fridge, cupboard or a drawer at work, you'll eat them. Only buy what you really need and no extras!

★ Men are motivated to lose weight for quite different reasons from women. Women usually want to lose weight so that they can look better in their clothes. However, it was clear from the male members of my trial team that they wanted to lose weight in order to improve their health. As the benefits to health will take some time to become apparent, men need to be motivated to get fit not just over the short term but to make lifestyle changes so that the benefits continue in the long term. It takes around 30 days to break a habit and to adopt a new one. Start today.

★ Keep temptation out of sight. Don't keep biscuits, chocolates, sweets and crisps at your work station. If you must have some at home for the other family members, then keep them well hidden from you.

★ To lose weight you need to eat around 1,700–2,000 calories a day (1,400 calories for women) and select foods that are low in fat. Check the nutrition labels on food products and try to only buy those with a maximum of four per cent fat.

★ Make the decision to become more active. If you like sport, consider joining a sports club or take regular lessons to improve your ability. Booking a series of lessons over a period of weeks will give you a regular commitment and will also encourage you to practise in between. As you see your performance improve you will be enouraged to continue. If you don't like sport, aim to become more active in your everyday life. Walk more, take the stairs more often and avoid lifts and escalators, put more energy into your gardening, lawn-mowing, hedge-cutting, and so on. See these activities as your workout and really enjoy the benefits.

★ Stop making excuses and putting off your diet and fitness campaign. There will never be an ideal time for you to diet – a time when there are no social engagements, business lunches or unplanned invitations. Life just isn't like that. If you do overindulge on food one day, don't worry. Just get back on track the next day and don't punish yourself.

★ Be realistic about your goals. Just as we can't change our height or our genes, neither can we change our bone structure or our basic physiological shape. We can however, do a heck of a lot to improve our appearance. Healthy eating and regular exercise can make us look and feel loads better. The benefits to health will greatly outweigh the few sacrifices you have to make.

★ Do keep a weekly record of your weight and inch loss progress (see page 271). It is also a good idea to have a photograph of yourself taken at the beginning of your weight-loss campaign. You will probably think this is a really lousy idea, but only by looking back at how you looked before, will you realise how much you have trimmed down. You don't have to show this photograph to anyone until you have lost your excess weight, but it will be a great record of how much you have achieved.

★ Try to be enthusiastic about your diet and fitness campaign. Be aware of the many benefits you will be enjoying within a few days of starting. There is no doubt that as my trial dieters lost weight their self-esteem improved, and even those men who said they didn't enjoy following the diet plan said they would definitely continue because they felt so much better.

★ Learn to cope with those difficult times when you just don't seem to be able to hold your willpower together – times when you have grossly overindulged or the scales show that you have gained a couple of pounds. This is very common and quite normal, so don't throw in the towel. Just get back on track the next day and put your misdemeanours behind you. Try and be more active over the next couple of days to compensate so that you get rid of those extra pounds quickly.

★ Picture yourself succeeding. Visualise yourself playing sport and not feeling tired at the end of it. Imagine yourself getting home after a tough day at the office and feeling ready to go for a run or play a game of sport instead of feeling drained and exhausted. Feel that you are totally in control of your life. The extraordinary thing is that the more we feel in control of our bodies, the more we are able to control our lives instead of everything else controlling us.

So don't starve yourself and don't punish yourself. Eat a healthy, calorie-controlled, low-fat diet, and be as active as possible. Exercise burns fat and makes you look and feel better. If you can start your day with 20 minutes of brisk walking or some other form of aerobic exercise, it will make all the difference to how you look and feel. Just do it. You will be really glad you did!

2

Tried and Tested

Devising a diet predominantly for men was a new adventure for me, so I decided to conduct a trial to put my theories to the test: namely that you could eat more calories than most diets would allow and drink three glasses of red wine a day (or any three units of alcohol) and still lose weight.

The trial diet was undertaken by 50 men of varying ages and occupations. Among them were managing directors, technical directors, consultants, accountants, police officers, a joiner, a carpenter, a sales rep, a civil engineer, catering managers and a casino inspector. I found my male volunteers via a number of sources: Marks & Spencer Head Office in Baker Street, London, The Leicester Mercury (my local newspaper), the Leicestershire Police Force, Leicestershire County Council, and Astra Chemicals at Loughborough. I also recruited some male members from Rosemary Conley Clubs and some of the women members' husbands.

The trial dieters were asked to follow the diet over a period of eight weeks and to fill in a questionnaire after that period. The diet that they were given was a much shorter version than the one in this book and included menus from both the Bachelor's Diet and the Gourmet Diet. Sixty-one per cent followed the diet on their own, while 39 per cent dieted with another person. Perhaps the most staggering result was that, over the eight-week period, 100 per cent of the trial dieters lost weight, with an *average* weight loss of 5.9kg (13lb) and an *average* reduction of 10cm (4in) from around the waist.

The greatest amount lost over the eight weeks was 12.7kg (24lb). This was achieved by Keith Houghton, a police officer from Leicestershire. The least amount lost, 0.9kg (2lb), was by Mr N. H. from Croydon. He did admit, however, that he hadn't stuck to the diet very strictly and that he'd eaten out five or six times a week, which had made dieting difficult. Nevertheless, he still lost 6cm (2.5in) from around his waist!

Prior to starting the diet, 17 per cent of my trial dieters described themselves as very overweight, 63 per cent as quite overweight, and only 20 per cent described themselves as slightly overweight.

Thirty per cent followed the diet strictly, 61 per cent moderately strictly, and nine per cent admitted to not following the diet strictly.

Ninety-six per cent said they wanted to reduce their weight around their waistlines, and when asked if they had managed to reduce this area on previous diets, 32 per cent said 'yes', 38 per cent said 'only a little' and 30 per cent said 'no' . I asked them if they were surprised with their inch losses on my diet. Fifty-four per cent said 'yes', 41 per cent said 'not particularly' and only four per cent said 'no'.

Ninety-six per cent of the trial dieters said they were pleased with the results they had achieved, and when asked which part of their body had reduced most significantly, the statistics came out as follows (they were invited to tick more than one option if they wished).

Seventy-two per cent said that their waists had reduced most significantly, and 51 per cent of these had also reduced their stomachs. Nine per cent said their thighs had reduced, six per cent said they had lost weight from their faces, and four per cent said that they had lost it off their hips. Four per cent lost weight off their chests, four per cent off their backsides and four per cent off their necks. Just two per cent found a reduction in the size of their arms.

When asked if they had enjoyed the diet (a rather courageous question on my part, I felt!) I am delighted to report that 52 per cent said they did. Thirty-nine per cent said 'no', while the others abstained – perhaps they were too polite to admit that 'enjoy' wasn't quite the right word. Despite the fact that 39 per cent said that they didn't enjoy following the diet, 91 per cent of the men said that they would make long-term lifestyle changes as a result of following the diet and felt significantly healthier after the eight-week eating programme.

I asked the dieters to undertake 30 minutes of physical activity at least three times a week. Seven per cent said that they exercised every day and another seven per cent said that they exercised almost every day. Thirty-three per cent said that they exercised three to four times a week, while 46 per cent said that they exercised once or twice a week. Only nine per cent admitted to taking no exercise at all.

It was clear to see from the completed questionnaires that those men who had exercised regularly definitely lost more weight and inches than those who didn't take regular exercise. There was a direct correlation between activity and rate of success. The more active the men were, the more weight they lost.

I was interested to know if their energy levels had increased as a result of eating a healthier diet and doing some exercise. Forty-six per cent said that their energy levels had improved, whereas 52 per cent said they had stayed the same and two per cent said that they had reduced.

Asked if they felt hungry on the diet, only 11 per cent said that they often felt hungry, and the remainder admitted to feeling hungry only very occasionally.

I've always believed that binge eating was more of a woman's problem than a man's, so I felt this was a golden opportunity to find out whether this was true. However, it appears that men do binge too, and 11 per cent of my trial dieters admitted to bingeing often prior to following the diet. Fifty-seven per cent admitted to bingeing occasionally, and only 33 per cent said that they had never binged. I then asked if they had binged while they were following the diet. None binged often, only 26 per cent binged occasionally and 74 per cent said that they didn't binge at all.

I asked what sacrifices they felt they had made as a result of following the diet and by far the winner in this category was chocolate, followed closely by crisps and cheese. The next thing my dieters missed most was biscuits, then cakes and butter. Other items that were mentioned were cream, puddings, pies, fish and chips, sweets, peanuts, olive oil, stew and dumplings, and pastries.

Christopher Barton from West Sussex listed his sacrifices as follows:

1 I love cheese and have had none.
2 Chips and crisps – out all together.
3 Cake – none except those with less than 4 grams of fat per 100 gram weight.

He added: 'I feel a strong sense of relief from losing the weight I was carrying around. I feel younger and much better looking and I do appear taller because I am less "boxy". My 112cm (44in) waist has gone down to 96.5cm (38in) and my belt is now being fastened five or six holes tighter. I am much livelier than before and more keen to tackle physical tasks.'

He also received some encouraging comments from those around him. One said: 'You look different – what have you done?' Another asked: 'Are you taller or something?' Chris, who has been attending a Rosemary Conley Club in Horsham regularly, commented: 'The 80 or so ladies with whom I have shared these events have been most encouraging and friendly, despite having their space invaded by this man in their midst.' In eight weeks, Christopher lost 8.2kg (18lb) and 20cm (8in) from his waist. A good result, indeed.

Eating out is always a potential problem when you are trying to lose weight. I asked how my dieters coped during the trial diet. Fifty-nine per cent said there was no problem, 41 per cent said that they didn't cope very well, but no one said that it was impossible.

I decided to find out more about the drinking habits of my team. What emerged was that my trial dieters varied from being teetotal to heavy drinkers, but even the heavy drinkers made some attempt to cut down while they were on the trial. Interestingly, providing they stuck to their three units of alcohol per day and spread these over the week rather than consuming their week's allowance in one go, what they drank had virtually no effect on their progress. They lost weight at about the same rate whether they drank wine, beer or spirits. Those who didn't drink at all lost virtually the same amount of weight as those who did drink. The difference between their results was negligible.

I was delighted to discover that 98 per cent of my trial dieters were non-smokers. With heart disease being such a massive killer and smoking such a high-risk factor, this was good news.

I wondered whether the diet would have any effect on the sex drive of the dieters. Seventy-two per cent said that there was either no improvement or no change, but 25 per cent admitted they had experienced a definite improvement (not everyone answered this question!).

When conducting a trial diet it is important to find out if the volunteers have been following a diet previously. Thirteen per cent had dieted prior to going on the trial and 87 per cent had not. This was, in fact, the first diet for 30 per cent of the volunteers, while 52 per cent said that, previously, they had dieted only very occasionally. Seventeen per cent admitted to going on more diets than they cared to remember.

When asked whether they were more successful on this diet than on previous ones, 67 per cent said 'yes' and 33 per cent said 'no'. I asked those who had answered 'yes' to tick the suggested reasons why this diet had been more successful (they were invited to tick more than one if they wished). Forty-two per cent said that they had greater success on this diet than on previous diets because it was easier to follow and involved no calorie counting. Thirty-six per cent said that they had greater willpower as a result of being part of a trial team, 34 per cent said that they could eat so much more on this diet than on most diets and that it offered more freedom of choice. Seventeen per cent said that it was quite different from any diet they had tried before and that they could have a drink and not feel guilty.

Seventy-two per cent of the dieters said that they now needed smaller-sized trousers, while 28 per cent found that the old ones were fitting better. Seventy-four per cent said that people had commented on their weight and inch losses, while 24 per cent said that no one had noticed.

I asked my dieters to indicate their level of self-confidence before the trial and how it might have improved afterwards. They were asked to score from 1–10. The results were quite interesting. Some men indicated that they felt no difference at all, while others felt their confidence had improved dramatically. Overall, an average of 10 per cent felt their confidence had increased.

Here are some of the comments that were made by the trial dieters.

Joe Mills from Surrey, who lost 5.4kg (12lb) and 11.5cm (4.5in) from his waist, wrote: 'People who had not seen me for a while automatically said, "You have lost a lot of weight." Now that the diet has finished, I find that I don't want to eat between meals and it feels normal to eat low-fat foods.'

Mr M. J. from Middlesex said that a couple of colleagues had asked jokingly, 'What happened to that fat bloke?' Simon Phillips from Kent said that his squash game had improved considerably. Dr M. S. from Leicestershire received comments such as 'You've lost weight and you look well!' after losing his 7.3kg (16lb) and 7.5cm (3in) from around his waist, and Alan Flavell from Leicestershire received comments such as 'You look good', 'You look really healthy' and 'That must be a good diet.' Alan lost 9.5kg (21lb) and 10cm (4in) from his stomach.

Mr J. P. from West Sussex said that this was the first diet that he had been on that made him feel substantially fitter as well as look better. He wrote: 'I shall keep going, as I know it's making a vast difference to my health.' He also received some encouragement from someone who commented, 'My goodness, you're losing weight. How did you manage it?'

Dennis Gatehouse from Surrey wrote to say that his asthma had improved and that he had much more stamina, as well as now having baggy trousers and a slimmer face. His work colleagues were so inspired by his success that they started dieting too. Dennis lost 8.2kg (18lb) and 10cm (4in) from around his waist.

Peter Dinallo from Surrey lost 10.4kg (23lb) and 10cm (4in) from around his waist. One person asked him: 'Have you lost weight? I thought your trousers were going to fall down!' Peter went on to say that his reduced waist measurement had given him greater mobility and that his improved fitness level had enabled him to work for longer periods. His blood pressure has lowered to 125/80, when previously it was up to 138/94. He continued: 'Improved comfort when riding my motorbike. When I have lost another stone I can get myself some new leathers.'

Brian McCarthy from Essex lost 11.3kg (25lb) and 10cm (4in) from his waist and reported a general feeling of increased alertness, energy and enthusiasm. His self-confidence level went from a score of 4 to 10, which was a dramatic improvement. One comment he received was, 'Where's your beer belly gone?' A similar comment was made to Mr B. P., who lost 3.6kg (8lb) on the trial diet in addition to the 4.1kg (9lb) he had already lost by attending a Rosemary Conley Club class. He also lost 11.5cm (4.5in) from around his waist during the trial. One friend commented: 'Your stomach has gone!' Mr R. A. from Leicestershire said that, after losing 4kg (9lb) and 7.5cm (3in) from his waist, he had lost his paunch.

Keith Houghton from Leicestershire lost 10.9kg (24lb) and 7.5cm (3in) from his waist. He received comments such as 'You look a lot better', 'How much have you lost?' and 'Which diet are you on? It must be a good one.' He wrote: 'This diet is by far the best I have been on. It was easy to follow, did not make me feel hungry and the results were far better than I imagined. In my opinion, a winner.'

So, a good result all round. Fifty happy trial dieters and lots of encouragement for you that it really works!

3

Your Very Good Health

I think many men are quite well informed about nutrition and often more concerned than their opposite sex about eating well for the sake of their health. We women tend to be more concerned about how we look rather than whether we will suffer a heart attack, in the same way that we are also more likely to exercise to improve our figures than to strengthen our hearts.

Anyone can pick up a leaflet in a pharmacy or the doctor's surgery on basic nutrition, but there are some real misunderstandings when it comes to certain foods and nutrients. First, let's look at cholesterol.

Cholesterol – it's not all bad news

Cholesterol has received enormous publicity over the past few years. Too much is bad for us; it can cause our arteries to 'fur up', which leads to heart disease. True, but that's not quite the full picture. In fact, small amounts of cholesterol are essential for our health and wellbeing. Without it, our bodies would not be able to function, because cholesterol is a necessary component of every cell in the body. It is found in large amounts in brain and nerve tissue and acts as a building block for various hormones, including the sex hormones testosterone, oestrogen and progesterone. It is also used to make bile acids, which are a vital part of digestion. So, cholesterol is not all bad news. The problems come when we have too much of it floating around in the bloodstream.

Cholesterol is a fatty substance that the body can make in the liver or we can take it from the food we eat. Cholesterol and other fatty substances such as triglycerides (fatty molecules formed in the liver from the fat we eat or from other internal sources) are insoluble in water. Think of trying to clean a greasy pan without using washing-up liquid – the fat congeals and floats to the surface. The body couldn't possibly cope with clumps of fat floating around, so cholesterol and triglycerides are dissolved within particles called lipoproteins and then carried to the tissues in the bloodstream. This is a very efficient system for getting these essential fatty substances to all the body's cells that need it.

There are three major types of lipoprotein:

1 *Very Low Density Lipoprotein (VLDL)*. VLDLs transport mainly triglycerides from the liver to the body's tissues. If you eat a lot of saturated fats, then you are likely to have lots of VLDLs floating around in your bloodstream. High triglyceride levels are known to be an important risk factor in heart disease.

2 *Low Density Lipoprotein (LDL)*. LDLs are the main transporters of cholesterol to your tissues. If your diet is high in cholesterol, your liver will manufacture more LDLs to handle it, which means your LDLs will

be high. So, LDLs are often termed the 'baddies', and high levels are a major risk factor in heart disease.

3 *High Density Lipoprotein (HDL)*. HDLs occur naturally in the body. They are the garbage collectors, picking up unused cholesterol in the blood, transporting it back to the liver for dismantling and converting into bile acids to help the digestive processes. A high level of HDLs is now thought to be very important for heart health, which is why HDLs are often termed the 'goodies'.

When you have your cholesterol checked, you are normally given a single value, say between 4 and 6 (the units are in millimoles per litre of blood) [mmol/l] and likely informed that an ideal value is around 5.2 mmol/l. This is a measure of your Total Cholesterol (TC). Basically, this is the total of your LDLs and HDLs. What these figures don't tell you is how much of this is bad LDL and how much is good HDL. Current research now tells us that, while high TC levels are not good for cardiovascular health, a high level of HDLs is a key preventer of heart disease. A low level of triglycerides (TG) is also highly desirable for coronary prevention.

Most certainly, diet can help control your blood lipids (fats), and that is why a low-fat, high-fibre eating plan is now routinely recommended. But exercise also has a very important part to play in controlling both cholesterol and triglycerides. Many studies have shown that regular aerobic exercise – at least 90 minutes per week – can considerably elevate your HDLs. In fact, most researchers consider that exercise is a more powerful factor than diet in raising HDLs. Other lifestyle

Cholesterol count

mmol/l	Desirable	Borderline	Abnormal
Total cholesterol	<5.2	5.2–7.8	>7.8
LDL cholesterol	<4.0	4.0–5.5	>5.5
HDL cholesterol	>1.0	0.9-1.0	<0.9

factors that can increase HDLs are weight control, not smoking and moderate alcohol consumption. Research has shown that exercise can also help lower triglyceride levels because the body uses triglycerides as a fuel for aerobic exercise. Total Cholesterol and LDLs are also shown to be lower in active people, largely due to their generally healthier lifestyles.

Controlling blood fat levels is a key feature in improving the health of our hearts. A combination of low-fat, high-fibre, healthy diet and regular aerobic activity is a powerful way of controlling cholesterol.

With clever marketing we are led to believe that a margarine low in saturated fat (and cholesterol) will prevent heart disease and we are tempted to believe that it will help our weight too. One of the most common misunderstandings comes from dieters who believe that spreading polyunsaturated margarine on their toast is helping their weight-loss campaign. A fine product though it is, it is not low in fat or calories. Butter contains 80 per cent fat, polyunsaturated margarines such as Flora, Olivio, Krona, Clover and Blueband have between 60 and 80 per cent, and olive oil, whether extra virgin or whatever, is a whopping 100 per cent fat – so don't be misled.

The only people to whom I would recommend polyunsaturated or monounsaturated margarines or oils are those who are slim and who have a history of heart disease in their family or who need to reduce their cholesterol levels but not their weight. For healthy, normal, slim people without hereditary risk factors, butter is natural and good in moderation. But if you want to lose weight, don't eat either, not even the low-fat, lower-calorie versions, as these are still high in fat.

New cholesterol-lowering foods containing plant stanol esters have appeared on the supermarket shelves. Stanol esters are natural substances which are extracted from certain plants and added to foods during their manufacture. These new cholesterol-lowering foods contain much higher levels of stanol esters than occur in the original plants. They have been sold in Scandinavia for many years but have only recently been introduced in Britain, firstly as a margarine and also as a cream cheese spread. These foods help to reduce cholesterol by blocking its absorption from the gut into the bloodstream. Three servings of foods enriched with stanol esters can reduce cholesterol absorption by about 30 per cent. The effect on blood cholesterol is not so dramatic, since many other factors determine blood cholesterol levels. However, research shows that people who use these foods regularly can decrease their blood cholesterol level by about 15 per cent over one year.

It is important to realise, though, that these foods specifically reduce the absorption of cholesterol – not total fat. They may help decrease blood cholesterol levels, but they won't help you to lose weight. Moreover, it is not yet clear exactly what effect this reduction in blood cholesterol may have on the chances of suffering from heart disease.

The nutrients for good health

Another misunderstanding is that we often associate foods that are healthy with foods that are boring. Well, it needn't to be that way.

It is important to eat a variety of foods to obtain the nutrients necessary for good health. I find it easier to think of nutrients as falling into two categories – tangible and intangible. Tangible nutrients are carbohydrates, proteins and fats. Minerals and vitamins fall into the intangible category because they are found *within* carbohydrates, proteins and fats. The key to good nutrition is getting the balance right. Eating too much of one thing can be as bad as eating too little of another. Here are some basic nutritional guidelines.

Carbohydrates

Carbohydrates include foods such as bread, rice, potatoes, pasta, cereals, as well as fruit and vegetables. These foods provide bulk in the diet and will only be stored as fat on the body if eaten in great excess. One gram of carbohydrate contains four calories. Carbohydrate should feature as the largest component in every meal, as out of all the food groups, it is the most important supplier of energy, and sixty per cent of the calories we consume each day should come from this food group.

Proteins

Proteins include foods such as meat, fish, poultry, eggs, cheese and milk. Their primary use is to help the body grow and to renew and repair existing tissues. Protein contains four calories per gram. It should be eaten in moderation, forming about a seventh of our daily calorie intake. Too much protein can be harmful because it has to be metabolised by the kidneys, so high-protein diets are not healthy or recommended. If we eat more protein than we need, the excess cannot be stored by the body. Instead, part of the protein will be excreted from the body and the remainder will be used to provide energy, therefore delaying the burning of fat.

Fats

Fats include foods such as oil, butter, margarine, cream and lard. Fat is also found in varying amounts in other foods such as meat and fish. It is a concentrated form of energy that is efficiently stored by the body for emergencies and also supplies some valuable nutrients for health. Fat contains nine calories per gram, which is more than twice the number of calories contained in carbohydrate or protein. On a weight-reducing diet, men should allow between 35 and 50 grams a day, while women should allow between 23 and 40 grams. When seeking to maintain weight, rather than trying to lose it, the maximum fat intake should not exceed 100 grams a day for men and 70 grams for women.

A small amount of fat is necessary for good health, and oily fish such as salmon, mackerel and herrings contain essential fatty acids that are particularly beneficial. For this reason I allow moderate amounts of oily fish on my diets.

Minerals

There are many minerals, all of which play an important role in helping us to achieve good health. In most cases, a varied and healthy diet will ensure we are not missing out. However, two important minerals – calcium and iron – deserve special mention. Since dairy products are the richest source of calcium and red meat is the richest source of iron, on a low-fat diet it is particularly important to make sure you are taking sufficient amounts. If you consume 300ml (½ pint) of skimmed or semi-skimmed milk each day (women may have 450ml/¾ pint), and eat red meat four times a week, you will probably meet your needs. Other good sources of iron are fortified breakfast cereals.

We need calcium to help maintain our bones and teeth and we need iron to make haemoglobin, which carries oxygen around the body in red blood cells. Too little iron and we become anaemic. Too little calcium and we are at high risk of developing osteoporosis. The tables that follow will help you check if you are getting enough of each nutrient. If you're not, you need to amend your diet accordingly.

Please note, these tables are intended as a rough guide only, since the iron and calcium content of foods may differ slightly for different cuts of meat and different brands of cereals, especially if they have been fortified.

Iron content of foods

Food	Serving size	mg
Liver	100g cooked weight	8
Kidney	100g cooked weight	7
Venison	100g cooked weight	8
Lean beef	100g cooked weight	3
Lean lamb	100g cooked weight	2

Pork	100g cooked weight	1
Ham	100g cooked weight	1
Duck	100g cooked weight	3
Chicken/turkey	100g cooked weight	1
Eggs	1	1
Chickpeas	100g cooked weight	3
Lentils	100g cooked weight	2.5
Baked beans	1 small can	2
Potatoes	100g cooked weight	0.5
Spinach	50g cooked weight	2
Watercress	50g	1
Cabbage	50g cooked weight	0.5
Broccoli	50g cooked weight	0.5
Dried fruit	50g	1
White bread	1 slice	0.8
Wholemeal bread	1 slice	0.8
Branflakes	25g	7 (fortified)
Weetabix	25g	4 (fortified)

The reference nutrient intake (RNI) for the male population is 8.7mg per day and 14.8mg per day for the female population.

Calcium content of food

Food	Serving size	mg
Milk	600ml	680
Cheddar cheese	25g	225
Cottage cheese	1 small pot	60
Yogurt	1 small pot	360
Eggs	1	25
Sardines	50g	250
Pilchards	50g	150

Prawns	50g	75
Tofu	100g	500
Ice-cream	50g	70
White bread	1 slice	30 (fortified)
Wholemeal bread	1 slice	7
Weetabix	25g	10
Shredded wheat	25g	12
Spinach	50g cooked weight	300
Watercress	50g	110
Dried fruit	50g	30

The reference nutrient intake (RNI) for both the male and female population is 700mg per day (800 mg per day for 15- to 18-year-old women).

Vitamins

Vitamins fall into two categories – fat-soluble and water-soluble. Vitamins A, D, E and K are fat-soluble and do not need to be consumed daily, since the body is able to store them. However, the B complex vitamins and vitamin C are water-soluble. As these cannot be stored by the body, they do need to be consumed daily. Each vitamin has its own special function and all are essential for good health.

Even though my diets are designed to be healthy and nutritionally balanced, I do recommend a multivitamin tablet daily, just to make doubly sure you have all the vitamins. This will ensure that you get all the micronutrients your body needs. The time-released type of vitamin tablet is best and they are widely available from health food stores and chemists. Always follow the recommended dose.

ACE advice

These days much attention has been focused on the antioxidant vitamins (vitamins A, C and E), which seem to reduce the risk of many serious diseases, including cancer and heart disease. The A of the ACE nutrients stands for beta-carotene, which is converted into vitamin A by the body. These vitamins help to zap the free radicals that occur naturally in the body in modest amounts.

For thousands of years the balance between antioxidants and free radicals in the body has been just fine, naturally. But now, with increased pollution, radiation from microwaves, mobile phones, TVs and computer screens, as well as increased exposure to stress and perhaps even pesticide residues and some drugs, the body is producing more free radicals. These are the 'bad guys'. To neutralise them we need to increase the number of antioxidants (the good guys) by eating more of the foods that contain the ACE vitamins. Some other nutrients also act as antioxidants, including minerals such as copper and zinc (found in meat), selenium (found in meat, fish, and cereals) and manganese (found mostly in tea).

In the right place, at the right time, free radicals have an important role to play. Think of them as nature's bleach. A small amount works wonders to kill germs, just as free radicals help to kill dangerous bacteria in the body. But in large amounts, or in the wrong places, free radicals (like bleach) can also cause great harm. They attack the body's own healthy cells, damaging cell membranes and leading to conditions as varied as cancer, premature ageing, cataracts and arthritis. They also have an effect on cholesterol in the blood, making it more likely to stick to the walls of the blood vessels and leading to heart disease. Antioxidants protect the body by neutralising these free radicals before they case any damage.

Fruit and vegetables are rich sources of natural antioxidants. Beta-carotene is easy to spot in foods – it is found in carrots (hence the name) and other red- and orange-coloured vegetables and fruits such as peppers, tomatoes, mangoes and papaya. Vitamin C is usually associated with citrus fruits such as oranges and grape-fruits, but blackcurrants and kiwi fruits are also rich sources. Potatoes, too, contain vitamin C, especially if you eat them in their skins. Vitamin E occurs naturally in many nuts and seeds, but we eat it mostly as either vegetable oils or in margarine (which is enriched in vit-amin E). On a low-fat diet vitamin E can be obtained from fortified breakfast cereals, dairy products and some dark green and red vegetables, such as spinach, peppers and carrots. Many other chemical compounds such as flavonoids, which occur naturally in some fruit and vegetables (particularly onions and apples), green tea, red wine (from the grape skins) and lycopenes (which make tomatoes and some other fruits turn red) also act as antioxidants.

Alcohol? Yes you can!

There is now good evidence that people who drink modest amounts of red wine each day live longer than those who are teetotal. In particular, it seems that wine can protect against heart disease. There are several rea-sons for this. First, alcohol helps to 'thin' the blood and prevent blood clotting. Secondly, wine leads to an increase in HDL (the 'good' cholesterol) and a decrease in LDL (the 'bad' cholesterol). Finally, the flavonoids found in wine act as antioxidants and decrease the risk of atherosclerosis (furring of the arteries). As flavonoids occur mainly in grape skins, they are found particularly in red wine but also in smaller concentrations in all kinds of wine. Another natural chemical found in wine, called phytoestrogen, has recently been linked to a reduced risk of breast cancer.

Some people enjoy a drink or two, but as soon as they start feeling any effect from it, they stop. Others, on the other hand, react quite differently. As soon as they get that feeling of crossing over the line, that the alcohol is taking over, they're off on a binge to get drunk. Only you know where you are on this scale and how alcohol affects your life and your relationships. Only you can make the decision to make changes if you feel you are addicted or dependent on alcohol. If so, please seek the help of your doctor or medical adviser.

If you want to lose weight but feel dependent on alcohol and unable to control your consumption, try abstaining completely while following this diet. It will give you a watershed to get yourself on track with your health. Eating healthily and taking regular exercise will all help you make a fresh start. If you are not alcohol-dependent and not-having-a-drink is just not an issue for you, you may find that having an occasional or regular (but not excessive) drink will help you both physically and psychologically.

There has been much discussion and many trials to determine the advantages and disadvantages of consuming alcohol, from whether it helps your heart to whether it makes you fat. It was even thought at one time that the calories from alcohol didn't count because the body processed calories from alcohol in a different way from other calories. But alcohol calories do count.

In its neat form, alcohol yields seven calories per gram, but of course we never consume alcohol in its pure state. It is always diluted by water, even in the strongest spirits. The calories in your favourite tipple may not always be directly related to the alcohol content, since many drinks also contain sugar, carbohydrates and sometimes even fat. A small glass of dry white wine or red wine contains around 95–100 calories. Sweeter wines have more calories because they contain additional carbohydrate.

Alcohol is easily absorbed by the stomach, but the only way the body can rid itself of alcohol is by burning it in the liver and other tissues. Since alcohol is essentially a toxin and the body has no useful purpose for storing it, the body prioritises the elimination of it at the cost of processing other foods you have eaten. Consequently, other foods may be converted to fat more readily than usual, thereby increasing your fat stores. So, if we drink wine with a meal it will delay the calories from the meal, especially those from fat, from being burned off.

In the trials that I ran before writing this book, those men who drank alcohol were no more and no less successful than those who didn't drink. In fact, the ones who did drink their three units of alcohol a day lost just as much weight as those that didn't. So, I have concluded that calories from the alcohol, providing they don't exceed 300 a day for men and 200 for women, are burned away without adversely affecting your weight loss progress – and that has to be good news!

The key is to have a little or a moderate amount each day, rather than drinking a lot on the occasional drinking binge. Perhaps one of the greatest dangers from drinking alcohol when you are dieting is that it is extremely effective at diluting your willpower. Because it's a relaxant, it's so easy to think 'Oh, what the heck, I'll diet tomorrow' and then really overindulge on the food front! Willpower really does dissolve in alcohol!

If you don't like red wine you can substitute any other form of alcoholic drink while following any of the diets in this book. However, do restrict your intake to three units a day (two for women) and familiarise yourself with the calorie values of each type of drink.

Reading nutrition labels

Nowadays most food products we buy contain lots of useful information on the nutrition label. This provides us with a breakdown of their nutritional content as well as the number of calories and amount of fat. To simplify matters, as far as weight control is concerned, the two key things to look at are the 'energy' and the 'fat' values.

The figure relating to 'energy' tells you the number of calories in 100 grams of the product (you can ignore the kJ figure which is used more frequently in other European countries – just look at the kcal one). You then need to calculate how much of the product you will actually be eating to work out the number of calories per portion. (see example on page 56).

Calorie content of alcoholic drinks

	Quantity	Calories
Bitter or pale ale	300ml (1/2 pint)	90
Brown ale	300ml (1/2 pint)	85
Light ale	300ml (1/2 pint)	75
Home brewed beers (all kinds)	300ml (1/2 pint)	120
Cider (dry)	300ml (1/2 pint)	100
Cider (vintage)	300ml (1/2 pint)	280
Lager	300ml (1/2 pint)	90
Lager (special brews)	300ml (1/2 pint)	200
Lager (alcohol free)	300ml (1/2 pint)	50
Martini (red)	single pub measure	80
Martini (white)	single pub measure	55
Port	25ml (1fl oz)	90
Sherry (cream)	50ml (2fl oz)	78
Sherry (dry)	50ml (2fl oz)	66
Spirits	single pub measure	50
Wine (dry white)	150ml (5fl oz) glass	95
Wine (sparkling white)	150ml (5fl oz) glass	110
Wine (rosé)	150ml (5fl oz) glass	100
Wine (dry red)	150ml (5fl oz) glass	100
Wine (sweet red)	150ml (5fl oz) glass	130

The fat content may be broken down into polyunsaturates and saturates, but, for anyone on a weight-reducing diet, it is the *total* fat content per 100 grams that is most relevant. I make the general and simple rule that my dieters should only select foods where the label shows the fat content as four grams or less per 100 grams weight of product, i.e. four per cent or less fat. I believe the actual amount of fat per portion is of lesser

Example

Nutritional information	
	Per 100g
ENERGY	172kJ/40kcal
PROTEIN	1.8g
CARBOHYDRATE	8.0g
(of which are sugars)	(2.0g)
FAT	0.2g
(of which are saturates)	(Trace)
FIBRE	1.5g
SODIUM	0.3g

importance. If you follow the simple four per cent rule and restrict your calorie intake to around 1,700–2,000 calories a day for men, and 1,400–1,600 calories a day for women, the fat content of your food will look after itself. The only exceptions to this rule are lean cuts of meat, lamb and pork which may be still just over the four per cent yardstick, and oily fish such as salmon, herrings and mackerel which may yield as much as 10 per cent fat, because of the other important nutrients they contain. Vegetarians may use the occasional drop of oil in the preparation of their food.

Remember that, although the four per cent rule is the ideal while you are trying to lose weight, I accept that there will be occasions when you might crave a high-fat treat or dine out and are unable to control what foods you eat. The occasional treat is not a disaster. The key is to enjoy it and not resort to a binge. Just try to balance the calories.

4

Cooking the Low-Fat Way

Cooking low fat is easier than you might think. It just takes a little bit of imagination. There are many low-fat foods that can be substituted for the high-fat ones you are probably used to using in your culinary exploits. In the next few pages, I will explain the benefits of using the appropriate implements and utensils, suggest which items are useful to have in your store cupboards and explain how to change your cooking techniques to enable you to make low-fat recipes that taste delicious. It will not take you long to automatically refrain from using olive oil – remember that it is 100 per cent fat – and discover that cooking with wine, garlic and herbs can still leave your tastebuds dancing.

Equipment you will need

Utensils

At one time, non-stick surfaces used to have a very short lifespan before becoming scratched and worn. Fortunately, in recent years, great progress has been made with non-stick pans, but the old adage 'you get what you pay for' still holds firm. Buy a cheap non-stick pan and the first time you slightly burn the pan, the surface will probably begin to peel.

It is worth investing in a top-quality, non-stick wok and frying pan, both with lids (Marks & Spencer has an excellent range that are strong and superb value). I use these two pans more than anything else in my kitchen. The lid is crucial, as it allows the contents of the pan to steam and this adds moisture to the dish.

Non-stick saucepans are useful, too, for cooking sauces, porridge, scrambled eggs and other foods that tend to stick easily. Lids are essential for these too.

Also, treat yourself to a set of non-stick baking tins and trays. Cakes, Yorkshire puddings, scones and lots more dishes can all be cooked the low-fat way.

When cleaning non-stick pans, always soak the pans first to loosen any food still inside. Then wash off with a non-abrasive sponge or cloth. Any brush or gentle scourer used carefully will do the trick of cleaning away every particle effortlessly without damaging the surface. Allowing pans to boil dry is the biggest danger with non-stick pans, so when cooking vegetables keep on eye on the water levels!

Non-scratch implements

Wooden spoons and spatulas, Teflon (or similar) coated tools and others marked as suitable for use with non-stick surfaces are a must. If you continue to use metal forks, spoons and spatulas, you will scratch and spoil the non-stick surface. Treat the surfaces kindly and good non-stick pans will last for years.

Other equipment

You will no doubt already have some of the items listed below, but there are some, such as baking parchment, that I find indispensable in a low-fat kitchen. However, it is neither necessary nor appropriate for you to have every item listed here unless you cook regularly for guests. Items in italics are ones that I consider essential.

Baking parchment
Aluminium foil
Kitchen paper
Measuring jugs (1 × ½ litre/1 pint), 1 × 1 litre/2 pint)
Kitchen scales (ones that weigh small amounts
   accurately)
Sieve (1 small, 1 large)
Colander (1 small, 1 large)
Flour shaker
Chopping boards (1 small, *1 medium*, 1 large)
Fish kettle (stainless steel)
Ovenproof dishes
Bowls (*1 × 1 litre/2 pints*, 1 × 2 litres/4 pints, 1 × 4
   litres/8 pints)
Plastic containers with lids
Ramekin dishes
Garlic press
Pastry brush
Whisk (balloon type)
Food processor
Good-quality can opener
Set of sharp knives (all sizes)
Palate knife

Pepper mill
Potato masher (non-scratch)
Pizza cutter
Pasta spoon (non-scratch)
Slotted spoon (non-scratch)
Lemon squeezer
Grater
Steamer
Wire rack (a grill rack is a good substitute)
Scissors
Multi-surface grater
Melon baller
Zester
Vegetable peeler
Juicer

Store cupboard

There are many items that are very useful to have in stock. Build up your store cupboard over a period of time to avoid a marathon shopping trip! All of these ingredients are allowed on a low-fat diet.

Arrowroot
Cornflour
Plain flour
Self-raising flour
Gelatine
Marmite
Bovril
Dried herbs
Tomato ketchup
HP Sauce

Fruity sauce
Barbecue sauce
Reduced-oil salad dressing
Balsamic vinegar
White wine vinegar
Black peppercorns
White pepper
Salt
Vegetable stock cubes
Chicken stock cubes
Beef stock cubes
Lamb stock cubes
Pork stock cubes
Long-grain easy-cook rice
Basmati rice
Pasta (various shapes and types)
Oats
Tabasco sauce
Soy sauce
Worcestershire sauce
Caster sugar
Brown sugar
Artificial sweetener

Fresh items
Garlic
Fresh herbs
Lemons
Oranges
Tomatoes
Eggs

Alternatives to cooking with fat

Low-fat cooking can be bland and dry, so it's important to add moisture and extra flavour to compensate for the lack of fat. Wine, water, soy sauce, wine vinegar, and even fresh lemon juice all provide liquid in which food can be 'fried' or cooked. Some thicker types of sauces can dry out too fast if they are added early on in cooking, so add them later when there is more moisture in the pan.

The art of dry-frying

I haven't used oil or butter in my frying for 13 years, yet I fry all the time. The secret of dry-frying is to have your non-stick pan over the correct heat. If it's much too hot, the pan will dry out too soon and the contents will burn. If the heat is too low, you lose the crispness recommended for a stir-fry. Practice makes perfect and a simple rule is to preheat the empty pan until it is hot (but not too hot) before adding any of the ingredients. Test if the pan is hot enough by adding a piece of meat or poultry. The pan is at the right temperature if the meat sizzles on contact. Once the meat or poultry is sealed on all sides (when it changes colour) you can reduce the heat a little as you add any other ingredients.

Cooking meat and poultry is simple, as the natural fat and juices run out almost immediately, providing plenty of moisture to prevent burning. When cooking minced meat I dry-fry it first and then place the meat in a colander to drain away any fat that has emerged. I then wipe out the pan with kitchen paper to remove any fatty residue before continuing to cook my shepherd's pie or bolognese sauce, or whatever. If you are using onions, always add them after you have dry-fried the meat and wiped out the pan or they will soak up the fat from the meat like a sponge.

Vegetables contain their own juices and soon release them when they become hot, so dry-frying vegetables works well too. When dry-frying vegetables it is important not to overcook them. They should be crisp and colourful so that they retain their flavour and most of their nutrients. Perhaps the most impressive results are obtained with onions. After a few minutes they go from being raw to translucent and soft and then on to become brown and caramelised. They taste superb and look for all the world like fried onions but taste so much better without all that fat.

Good results are also obtained when dry-frying large quantities of mushrooms, as they sweat and make lots of liquid. Using just a few mushrooms produces a less satisfactory result unless you are stir-frying them with lots of other vegetables. If you are using just a small quantity, therefore, you may find it preferable to cook them in vegetable stock.

Flavour enhancers

Adding freshly ground black pepper to just about any savoury dish is a real flavour enhancer. You need a good pepper mill and, ideally, you should buy your peppercorns whole and in large quantities. Ready ground black pepper is nowhere near as good. I find it sandy and tasteless, so give this one a miss.

When cooking rice, pasta and vegetables, add a vegetable stock cube to the cooking water. Although stock cubes do contain some fat, the amount absorbed by the food is negligible and the benefit in flavour is noticeable. I always save the cooking water from vegetables to make soups, gravy and sauces. Again, the fat from the stock cube, divided between however many portions I am serving, is very small.

When making sandwiches, spread sauces such as Branston, mustard, horseradish and low-fat dressings straight on the bread. This helps the inside of the sandwich to stay 'put' and, because all these items are quite highly flavoured, you won't miss the butter. Do make sure you use fresh bread, though, for maximum taste.

Here is a quick reference list of ingredients or cooking methods that can be substituted for traditional high-fat ones.

Cheese sauces Use small amounts of low-fat Cheddar, a little made-up mustard and skimmed milk with corn-flour.

Custard Use custard powder and follow the instructions on the packet, using skimmed milk and artificial sweetener in place of sugar to save more calories.

Cream Instead of double cream or whipping cream, use 0% fat Greek yogurt or fromage frais. Do not boil. Instead of single cream, use natural or vanilla-flavoured yogurt or fromage frais.

Cream cheese Use quark (skimmed soft cheese).

Creamed potatoes Mash potatoes in the usual way and add fromage frais in place of butter or cream. Season well.

French dressing Use two parts apple juice to one part wine vinegar, and add a teaspoon of Dijon mustard.

Marie Rose Dressing Use reduced-oil salad dressing mixed with tomato ketchup and a dash of Tabasco sauce and black pepper. (See also recipe on page 259.)

Mayonnaise Use fromage frais mixed with two parts cider to one part lemon juice, plus a little turmeric and sugar, or buy a branded low-fat version and use sparingly. (See also recipe on page 256.)

Porridge Cook with water the night before it is required. Make to a sloppy consistency, cover and leave overnight. Reheat before serving and serve with cold milk and sugar or honey.

Roux Make a low-fat roux by adding dry plain flour to a pan containing the other ingredients and 'cooking off' the flour, then add liquid to thicken. Alternatively, use cornflour mixed with cold water or milk, bring to the boil and cook for 2–3 minutes.

Thickening for sweet sauces Arrowroot, slaked in cold water added to fruit juice and brought to the boil, is good because it becomes translucent when cooked.

Stocks

Any restaurant chef will tell you that the secret of a good sauce relies on a very good stock. Home-made stock is very time-consuming to make but well worth the effort, as the final flavours are quite different from any convenient stock cube alternatives. If you do decide to make your own stock, be sure to chill it completely. This allows the fat to set, making it easy to remove and discard before adding the stock to your cooking.

There are four basic stocks which are used as a base for many dishes. White stock is pale and light and made from meat and poultry. Unbrowned beef and chicken are excellent for this purpose, while lamb, pork and duck contain much higher levels of fat. Brown stock is made by browning the meat or bones first – you can either dry-fry the meat in a non-stick pan or roast in a hot oven (the latter method gives a darker colour). Both white and brown stock are then flavoured with root vegetables such as carrots, celery, onions and leeks and left to simmer in plenty of water for 1½–2 hours. A brown stock may be coloured with tomato purée or gravy browning for a deep finish.

Fish stock is quite different and needs careful cooking. The stock should not be allowed to simmer for more than 20 minutes or the bones will make the stock bitter. You can use the bones, heads, skin and tails of any white fish such as sole, brill or plaice. Avoid fatty fish such as mackerel, which will make the stock oily.

Vegetable stock can be made easily by simmering a wide selection of fresh vegetables, taking care not to overpower the flavour with one particular ingredient. You can add tomato purée for additional flavour.

Many recipes in this book use stock cubes for convenience and it is well worth spending a little extra on the better quality ones. Generally, one stock cube will make up with 600ml (1 pint) of water.

Salad dressings

The secret of a good salad is in the dressing. We are so used to being served oily dressings that they become something of a habit. The key is to learn how to make a good dressing without using oil, and it really isn't that difficult. Try it, and you'll be amazed how quickly your tastebuds adapt. Once you've followed a low-fat diet for any length of time, you'll find the taste of oil becomes extremely unpalatable. Here are some ideas for low-fat or fat-free dressings.

★ Balsamic Dressing (see recipe, page 256).
★ Fat-free Mayonnaise (see recipe, page 256).
★ Honey and Orange Dressing (see recipe, page 257).
★ Oil-Free Vinaigrette (see recipe, page 258).
★ Garlic and Yogurt Dressing (see recipe, page 257).
★ Marie Rose Dressing (see recipe, page 259).

5

The Red Wine Diet

The right eating plan for you is the one that works for YOU. If you want to have your main meal at lunchtime, that's fine. If you want to save some calories from breakfast and lunch and have a three- or four-course banquet at night, that's fine too. Try to avoid skipping meals completely, or you will be tempted to start snacking later.

I don't think it's crucial that you don't eat late at night, so long as it's not a large meal. Breakfast is a must, though, even if you don't eat it until 10am. Eating breakfast kick-starts your metabolism and gets things moving in your body. During the night your body is a digesting-and-mending machine. Imagine it has a day and a night shift. The night-shift workers come on duty when you go to bed, and carry out lots of repairs and maintenance while you are asleep. All the day's food is broken down and the nutrients distributed where they are needed. By the morning, the work is complete, so by getting up and having a fresh delivery of food (breakfast) you give the signal to the maintenance night shift to leave and rest while the day-shift workers, the energy-makers, wake up and take over. Their job is to ensure that the energy values of the foods you eat during the day are available as and when you need them. This is why breakfast is so important.

Now select the diet most suited to you.

Diet 1: The No Diet Diet (page 70)

This is for those who are prepared to make some changes to their eating patterns but who don't want to follow a diet plan. If you choose this one, you will lose weight but not as much as you would on one of the other diet plans.

Diet 2: The Bachelor's Diet (page 74)

This diet is for men (and women) who live alone and don't want to peel potatoes and chop onions but are happy to heat up a ready-made meal in a microwave. In addition, you can select any meal from the Gourmet Diet menus. (Women should check their calorie allowance on pages 23–25 and the calorie allocation per meal.)

Diet 3: The Gourmet Diet (page 87)

This one is for people who like to cook, or who have someone to cook for them. In addition, you can substitute any item from the Bachelor's Diet. (Women should reduce the portion sizes by 25 per cent.)

The No Diet Diet

If you want to lose weight but you really don't want to follow a diet plan, then just follow these simple rules and you will lose weight, but you may not lose it as fast as you would on one of the other diet plans.

HERE ARE THE DOs

1 DO eat three moderate-sized meals a day – breakfast, lunch and dinner.

2 DO limit your alcohol consumption to three units of alcohol per day, preferably three glasses of red wine, but if you wish you can drink 3×300ml ($3 \times \frac{1}{2}$ pint) measures of lager or beer, or three single measures of spirit plus slimline mixers.

3 DO look at the nutrition labels on every item of food before you buy it. Only purchase those products that contain 4 grams or less fat per 100 grams of product (i.e. 4 per cent fat).

4 DO increase your activity levels. At every opportunity be more energetic. Use the stairs more, walk further and more often. Try the progressive jogging programme on page 121.

5 DO cut out all visible fat from your diet. That includes butter, margarines, Flora, Olivio, low-fat spreads, oil, olive oil, lard, dripping, cream, crème fraîche, French dressing, mayonnaise, and so on. It will take a couple of weeks to get used to eating food without added fat, but after a month you won't want it, anyway, when you see how many inches you've lost!

6 DO eat a dessert if you want to. Just select low-fat

(max. 4 % fat) puddings. Avoid those made with pastry, cream, chocolate and cheese.

7 DO eat enough at mealtimes to fill you up, otherwise you might be tempted to eat between meals. Vegetables are great fillers with your main meal.

8 DO eat three pieces of fruit a day. These can be eaten at any time.

9 DO drink 300ml ($\frac{1}{2}$ pint) semi-skimmed milk each day – in teas, coffees and on your cereal. You can have skimmed milk if you prefer, but it is an acquired taste!

10 DO drink as much water as possible. Diet drinks are also unrestricted.

11 DO continue to dine out, but avoid anything fried, coated in breadcrumbs or batter or cooked in pastry. Choose a jacket potato or boiled potatoes in preference to chips. Ask for your food to be cooked without fat and have fat-free dressings on salads.

12 DO choose soup as a starter – it is a good filler. Choose consommé or vegetable-based soups rather than creamy ones, but forget the bread roll.

13 DO weigh yourself and measure your waist every week at the same time of day under the same conditions – same scales, no clothes, in the morning, etc. Keep a record of your progress on page 271.

14 DO balance the effects of a sumptuous meal out by taking extra exercise the next day.

15 DO cook and serve all food without adding fat.

AND THE DON'Ts

1 DON'T nibble between meals.
2 DON'T buy any chocolate or sweets.

3 DON'T save up your daily alcohol allowance and drink it all in one go.

4 DON'T skip meals.

5 DON'T eat just one massive meal a day.

6 DON'T eat biscuits, cakes, pastries – in fact, anything with more than 4% fat content, except oily fish.

7 DON'T eat any of the foods listed below.

Foods to avoid

The following foods are strictly forbidden while you are trying to lose weight on the No Diet Diet, unless they are available in brands that contain 4% or less fat.

Avocado pears
Black pudding
Butter
Butterscotch
Cakes
Cheese (all varieties except cottage cheese)
Chocolates
Chocolate spread
Cocoa and cocoa products
Crackers
Cream
Cream cheese
Cream from full-fat milk
Crème fraîche
Crème caramel
Crisps (including low-fat crisps and snacks)
Dressings and sauces containing more than 4% fat
Drinking chocolate
Dripping

Egg custard
Faggots
Fatty meats (e.g. goose)
Fried foods of any kind (except dry-fried)
Fudge
Haggis
Horlicks
Lard
Low-fat spreads
Lemon curd
Mayonnaise
Marzipan
Olives
Pastries
Pâté
Quiches
Salami
Scotch eggs
Soured cream
Sponge puddings
Suet
Yogurt (full fat), including Greek yogurt (except
   Total 0%)

The freedom given to you in this diet is compensated by the strict guidelines on pages 70–73. If you stick to these guidelines you will lose weight and inches. If you cheat, you may not and you may be better suited to one of the more formal eating plans that follow.

The Bachelor's Diet

If you don't like cooking, or simply don't have the time, this diet contains lots of suggestions for quick and easy low-fat menus and ready-made meals.

First calculate your personal daily calorie allowance. To do this, look at the charts on pages 70–75. Check what your total energy requirement is likely to be by looking at the figure listed alongside your weight in the correct age category and under the heading that most accurately describes your activity level. Knock off 900 calories to create a sufficient deficit to effect a good rate of weight loss. Hopefully, the number of calories you will be burning by taking *additional* exercise will average 200 per day, and this will then create the 1,100 calorie deficit you need each day to achieve a weight loss of approximately 1kg (2lb) per week. Now enter your daily calorie allowance here:

My calorie allowance is _____

If your allowance is more than 2,000 calories per day, you can add additional calories by eating more fruit. If your daily allowance is less than 2000 calories, do not have the treat allowed in this diet. Also, as you lose weight you may wish to recalculate and reduce your calories if you continue with your weight-loss programme. (Women should check their calorie allowance on page 23–25 and the calorie allocation per meal – see opposite.)

Select one breakfast, one lunch, one dinner and dessert, plus one treat each day, adding additional treats or increasing your portion sizes to bring your daily total up to your allowance. If you wish, you can select menus or recipes from the Gourmet Diet or even make up your own menu selection, providing you keep within your calorie allowance and select foods with a maximum of 4% fat.

For good health you should consume five helpings of fruit and/or vegetables daily, so try to incorporate these within your menu selections.

Here is a reminder of a typical daily calorie allocation. Remember, you can substitute any three units of alcohol (two for women) for the red wine, e.g. 3 × 300ml (3 × ½ pint) measures of beer or lager, 3 single measures of spirits with slimline mixers.

	Men	Women
Breakfast	300 kcal	225 kcal
Lunch	450 kcal	300 kcal
Dinner	500 kcal	375 kcal
Dessert	100 kcal	75 kcal
Treats	200 kcal	Nil
300ml (½ pint) of skimmed or semi-skimmed milk (450ml/¾ pint for women)	150 kcal	225 kcal
3 glasses red wine	300 kcal	
2 glasses red wine		200 kcal
TOTAL	2000 kcal	1400 kcal

Diet notes

★ 1 piece fresh fruit means 1 average apple, orange etc., or 115g (4oz) of any fresh fruit.

★ For guidance, 1 slice regular bread from a large, thin-sliced loaf weighs 25g (1oz). A slice from a large, medium-sliced loaf weighs 40g (1½oz).

★ Unlimited vegetables includes all vegetables, except potatoes, providing they are cooked and served without fat.

★ For sauces and dressings check the nutrition panel on the label before you buy and only select those with 4 grams or less fat per 100 grams of product, except for items such as mustard of which you will consume only minimal amounts.

Breakfasts

Approx. 300 kcal. (Women should reduce quantities by approximately 25 per cent)

★ 50g (2oz) any cereal with milk (in addition to allowance) and 2 teaspoons sugar, plus 1 piece fresh fruit.

★ 50g (2oz) [dry weight] porridge cooked in water the night before. Serve with milk (in addition to allowance) and 2 teaspoons sugar or honey.

★ 5 pieces any fresh fruit.

★ 25g (1oz) any cereal with milk (in addition to allowance), plus 1 teaspoon sugar, plus 1 medium slice wholemeal toast, spread with 2 teaspoons marmalade, honey or preserve.

★ 1 dry-fried or poached egg, 2 St Michael 95% Fat Free Chipolata Sausages, 4 tomatoes, halved and grilled, 115g (4oz) mushrooms cooked in stock without fat, plus 1 medium slice wholemeal toast.

★ 2 medium slices wholemeal toast topped with 175g (6oz) baked beans and 2 grilled tomatoes.

★ 1 whole grapefruit, 1 poached or boiled egg, and 2 slices wholemeal toast spread with Marmite.

★ 2 bananas plus 200g (7oz) low-fat yogurt, any flavour.

★ Bacon sandwich: 2 rashers lean back bacon, grilled with all visible fat removed, placed between 2 slices wholemeal bread spread with brown sauce, ketchup or mustard.

★ 2 Weetabix plus 150ml (¼ pint) milk (in addition to allowance) and 2 teaspoons sugar.

★ 2 Shredded Wheat plus 150ml (¼ pint) milk (in addition to allowance) and 2 teaspoons sugar.

★ 3 grilled turkey rashers, 1 slice wholemeal toast topped with 175g (6oz) baked beans, plus 2 large grilled tomatoes.

★ ½ melon, 225g (8oz) grapes and 200g (7oz) low-fat yogurt.

★ 2 medium slices wholemeal bread spread with mustard (optional) filled with 75g (3oz) wafer thin ham.

★ 2 slices toast spread with marmalade (no butter or margarine).

★ 65g (2½oz) any cereal plus extra 150ml (¼ pint) milk (in addition to allowance).

★ Fresh Fruit Smoothy (see recipe, page 158).

Lunches

Approx. 450 kcal. (Women should reduce serving sizes by a third, i.e. to 300 kcal.)

★ 1 × 340g pack St Michael 95% Fat Free Haddock with Mustard Sauce and Rice, plus 2 pieces fresh fruit.

★ 1 × 280g pack St Michael 95% Fat Free Filled Plaice Supreme, plus 1 Pot Light Pasta Snack.

★ 1 × 450g pack St Michael 95% Fat Free Bouill-abaisse, plus 40g (1½oz) bread and 1 × 150g (5oz) pot low-fat yogurt or 1 piece fresh fruit.

★ 1 × 115g pack St Michael 95% Fat Free Mushroom Pâté, plus 50g (2oz) bread or toast.

★ ½ pack St Michael 95% Fat Free Ready to Eat Tomato and Basil Chicken Fillets, or Chicken Tikka, or Chinese Style Chicken, plus large mixed salad with fat-free dressing, and 50g (2oz) bread.

★ 1 pack St Michael Tagliatelle with Ham and Mush-room, plus 1 St Michael 95% Fat Free Mousse and 1 apple or pear.

★ 1 pack St Michael 95% Fat Free Healthy Choice sandwiches (choose from Bacon, Lettuce and Tomato, Tuna and Tomato, Smoked Turkey and Coleslaw, or Smoked Ham), plus 1 × 150g pot St Michael 95% Fat Free Extremely Fruity Bio Yogurt or 2 pieces fresh fruit.

★ 1 pack St Michael 95% Fat Free Healthy Choice Chicken Tikka Sandwich, plus 1 St Michael 95% Fat Free Mousse and 1 banana.

★ 1 St Michael 95% Fat Free Jacket Potato with Chilli, plus 1 St Michael 95% Fat Free Mousse and 1 banana.

★ 1 St Michael 95% Fat Free Jacket Potato deep filled with Tuna and Sweetcorn, plus 1 St Michael 95% Fat Free Mousse and 1 banana.

★ 1 × 400g pack Asda Quorn Sweet and Sour Egg Fried Rice, plus 1 apple or pear.

★ 1 pack Knorr Taste Breaks Tomato and Mozzarella Pasta, plus 1 apple or pear.

★ 1 McVitie's Go Ahead Pizza Square, plus salad with fat-free dressing, and 2 pieces fresh fruit.

★ 1×340g pack Linda McCartney Chilli Con Carne, plus large salad with fat-free dressing, 1×150g (5oz) pot low-fat yogurt and 1 piece fresh fruit.

★ 1×340g pack Linda McCartney Ploughman's Pie, plus large salad with fat-free dressing, and 1 piece fresh fruit.

★ 1×320g pack Linda McCartney Lasagne, plus large salad with fat-free dressing, and 1 low-fat yogurt.

★ 1×300g pack Tesco 95% Fat Free Lasagne, plus large salad with fat-free dressing, and 2 pieces fresh fruit.

★ 1×400g pack Tesco Chicken in White Wine, plus large salad with fat-free dressing, and 1×150g (5oz) pot low-fat yogurt.

★ 1×400g tin HP Pasta Menus Vegetable Lasagne, plus 50g (2oz) French bread and 1 low-fat yogurt.

★ 1 Sainsbury's Fresh 'n' Ready Pasta Pomodoro Meals in Minutes, plus 50g (2oz) French bread and 1 piece fresh fruit.

★ 1 Sainsbury's Noodle Recipes (choose from Vegetable, Chicken, Beef, or Tomato and Herb), plus 1×150g (5oz) pot low-fat yogurt.

★ 1 Sainsbury's Noodle Recipes (choose from Tomato and Herb or Cheese and Broccoli), plus 50g (2oz) bread and 1 piece fresh fruit.

★ 1 Sainsbury's Noodle Recipes Chicken Chow Mein, plus 1×150g (5oz) pot low-fat yogurt and 1 piece fresh fruit.

★ 1 Sainsbury's Noodles Recipes Hot and Spicy.

★ 1 Sainsbury's Noodles Recipes Thai Chicken, plus 1 piece fresh fruit.

★ 1 St Michael 95% Fat Free Ham and Mushroom Pizza, plus large salad with fat-free dressing.

★ 1 St Michael 95% Fat Free Chargrilled Vegetable Pizza, plus large salad with fat-free dressing.

★ Vegetable Croquettes (see recipe, page 176), served with Branston pickle, plus large salad with fat-free dressing.

★ Pasta with Spinach Sauce (see recipe, page 176), plus large salad with fat-free dressing, and 1 piece fresh fruit.

Dinners

Approx. 500 kcal. (Women should reduce portion sizes by approximately 25 per cent.)

★ 1 × 227g pack St Michael 95% Fat Free Cod and Broccoli Bake, plus 50g (2oz) [dry weight] pasta, and 50g (2oz) French bread.

★ 1 × 300g pack St Michael 95% Fat Free Tuna and Sweetcorn Pie, plus 50g (2oz) [dry weight] pasta, large salad with fat-free dressing.

★ 1 × 300g pack St Michael 95% Fat Free Salmon Pie, plus 175g (6oz) potatoes and unlimited other vegetables.

★ 1 × 300g St Michael 95% Fat Free Roast Chicken Pie, plus 225g (8oz) potatoes and unlimited other vegetables.

★ 1 × 600g pack St Michael 95% Fat Free Creamy Chicken and Ham with Rice, plus small salad with fat-free dressing.

★ ½ × 500g pack St Michael 95% Fat Free Moroccan Chicken Tagine, plus 50g (2oz) [dry weight] rice and unlimited vegetables, excluding potatoes.

★ 1×454g pack St Michael 95% Fat Free Chicken with Mushrooms in a Red Wine Sauce, plus 115g (4oz) boiled potatoes, and salad with fat-free dressing.

★ 1×350g pack St Michael 95% Fat Free Chicken, Tomato and Basil, plus 175g (6oz) potatoes and unlimited other vegetables.

★ 1×400g pack St Michael 95% Fat Free Chicken Chow Mein, plus 50g (2oz) French bread.

★ 1 whole pack St Michael 95% Fat Free Chinese Menu for Two. (This two-pack serving contains 615 calories. If you want to eat it all, you can, but NO PUDDING afterwards, please!)

★ 1×440g pack St Michael 95% Fat Free Moroccan Lemon Chicken, plus 115g (4oz) potatoes and unlimited other vegetables.

★ 1×325g Asda Healthy Choice 98% Fat Free Quorn Fillets roasted in Pepper Sauce, plus 225g (8oz) potatoes and unlimited other vegetables.

★ 1×325g pack Asda Quorn Fillets in White Wine Sauce, plus 225g (8oz) potatoes and unlimited other vegetables.

★ 1×400g pack Asda Quorn Tikka Masala with Rice.

★ 1×450g pack Asda Healthy Choice Chicken For-restière, plus 115g (4oz) potatoes and salad with fat-free dressing.

★ 1×500g pack Asda Mussels and Bacon in a Beer Sauce, plus 50g (2oz) French bread.

★ 1×368g pack Bird's Eye Healthy Option 95% Fat Free Chicken Tikka Masala, plus large salad with fat-free dressing.

★ 1 × 320g pack Weight Watchers from Heinz Chicken Hotpot, plus 175g (6oz) potatoes and unlimited other vegetables.

★ 1 × 300g pack Weight Watchers from Heinz Lamb Moussaka, plus 115g (4oz) French bread and a small salad with fat-free dressing.

★ 1 × 350g pack Sainsbury's Fresh 'N' Ready Mushroom Risotto Meals in Minutes, plus salad with fat-free dressing.

★ 1 × 450g pack Sainsbury's 95% Fat Free Be Good to Yourself Prawn Kadai with Pilau Rice.

★ 1 × 450g pack Sainsbury's 95% Fat Free Be Good to Yourself Tagliatelle with Chicken, Tomato & Basil, plus salad with fat-free dressing.

★ 1 × 450g pack Sainsbury's 95% Fat Free Be Good to Yourself Sweet and Sour Chicken with Egg Fried Rice (this meal contains 608 calories, so no pudding please!).

★ 1 × 450g pack Sainsbury's 95% Fat Free Be Good to Yourself Gemellia Pasta with Salsa & Bacon, plus large salad with fat-free dressing.

★ 1 × 450g pack Sainsbury's 95% Fat Free Be Good to Yourself Tagliatelle with Ham and Mushroom, plus large salad with fat-free dressing.

★ 1 × 450g pack Sainsbury's 95% Fat Free Be Good to Yourself Roasted Vegetable Cannelloni, plus small salad with fat-free dressing.

Desserts

Approx. 100 kcal. (Women should reduce quantities by approximately 25 per cent.)

★ 225g (8oz) fresh fruit.

★ 1 pot any low-fat yogurt up to 100 kcal.

★ Any St Michael 95% Fat Free Mousse.

★ 1 × 100ml pot Weight Watchers from Heinz 95% Fat Free Iced Dessert.

★ 1 serving Tesco Sorbet – lemon, mango or blackcurrant.

★ 1 scoop Weight Watchers from Heinz Toffee Fudge Swirl.

★ 1 serving Wall's 'Too Good To Be True' iced dessert.

★ 1 Sainsbury's Be Good to Yourself 96% fat free Raspberry Mousse.

★ 1 × 90g pot St Ivel Shape Summer Fruit Torte – Summer Fruits or Exotic Fruits.

★ 1 serving Sainsbury's 95% Fat Free Be Good to Yourself Vanilla Ice-cream.

★ 1 × 130g tin Sainsbury's Fruit Cocktail in Light Syrup.

★ Hot Cherries (see recipe, page 240).

★ 1 × 100g serving any fruit cocktail in fruit juice, topped with 1 low-fat fromage frais or yogurt with no more than 50 kcal.

★ 1 meringue nest filled with 115g (4oz) any fresh fruit, topped with 1 tablespoon low-fat fromage frais.

★ 1 Weight Watchers from Heinz Chocolate Mousse, plus 1 apple.

★ 75g (3oz) fresh pineapple rings topped with 50g (2oz) pineapple-flavoured low-fat fromage frais.

★ 1 × 50ml serving Wall's 'Too Good To Be True' strawberry iced dessert topped with 115g (4oz) fresh strawberries.

★ 1 × 110g pot St Ivel Shape dessert.

★ 1×70g pot Nestlé Aero Super Light Chocolate Mousse.
★ 1×125g pot Provamel Chocolate or Vanilla Soya Dessert with Added Calcium.

Treats

Approx. 200 kcal (men only).

★ 2×St Michael 95% Fat Free Crispie Cakes.
★ 1×⅙th serving St Michael 95% Fat Free Strawberry Cheesecake.
★ 1 St Michael 95% Fat Free Apricot Flapjack.
★ 1 slice St Michael 95% Fat Free Orange and Lemon Drizzle Cake.
★ 1 St Michael 95% Fat Free Orange and Chocolate Sponge Cake.
★ 1×⅙th serving St Michael 95% Fat Free Orange and Passion Fruit Cake.
★ 1×90g serving Tesco Low-Fat Mandarin Cheesecake.
★ 1×⅙th serving Tesco Coffee Dessert Cake.
★ 1 serving Tesco Chocolate and Toffee Cake.
★ 1 serving Tesco 95% Fat Free Lemon and Orange Cake.
★ 1 Weight Watchers from Heinz Chocolate Tiramisu.
★ 1 Weight Watchers from Heinz Chocolate and Toffee Dessert.
★ 1 serving McVitie's Go Ahead 95% Fat Free Blackcurrant Cheesecake.
★ 1 serving Sainsbury's Be Good to Yourself 98% fat free Lemon Curd Swirl.
★ Any 95% fat free yogurt up to 200 kcal.

★ 4 pieces or 450g (1lb) any fresh fruit.

★ 50g (2oz) bread.

★ 50g (2oz) [dry weight] rice or pasta added to any meal of your choice.

★ 2 thin slices Soreen Fruit Malt Loaf (no butter!).

★ 1 × 250g pack John West Tuna Light Lunch – Tomato Salsa or Mediterranean or French Style.

Eating out

Pub food

★ Soup and roll, plus 1 round of sandwiches (no butter or margarine) spread with horseradish sauce or mustard and filled with sliced beef or ham.

★ Grilled fillet steak with small jacket potato (no butter), served with salad (no dressing).

★ Grilled salmon with new potatoes, vegetables or salad (no dressing).

Restaurant food

★ Melon to start, then grilled steak or fish or chicken served with boiled potatoes (served without butter), unlimited vegetables or salad (ask for a low-fat dressing), followed by a sorbet or a fresh fruit dessert.

★ Vegetable soup (no bread roll). Select any main course cooked without fat and a low-fat dessert.

★ Melon cocktail, followed by grilled fish, boiled potatoes and unlimited vegetables (no butter) plus tartare sauce or ketchup. A dessert such as pears in red wine would be a good choice.

★ Prawn cocktail or smoked salmon or soup (no bread) to start, followed by grilled steak (no fat), with 1 jacket potato and salad (with a low-fat dressing dressing), plus a sorbet for dessert.

★ Roast chicken, beef or lamb, served with boiled vegetables including potatoes (no butter) and gravy, plus ice-cream or fruit salad.

★ Grilled fish (any kind), served with boiled vegetables including potatoes (no butter), plus ice-cream or fruit salad.

The Gourmet Diet

This extensive diet is designed for the man who enjoys cooking or entertaining or has someone to share mealtimes with.

The calorie allowance for this diet is the same as for the Bachelor's Diet and is allocated as follows. Remember, you can substitute any three units of alcohol (two for women) for the red wine, e.g. 3×300ml ($3 \times \frac{1}{2}$ pint) measures beer or lager, 3 single measures of spirits with slimline mixers.

	Men	Women
Breakfast	300 kcal	225 kcal
Lunch	450 kcal	300 kcal
Dinner	500 kcal	375 kcal
Dessert	100 kcal	75 kcal
Treats	200 kcal	Nil
300ml ($\frac{1}{2}$ pint) of skimmed or semi-skimmed milk (450ml/$\frac{3}{4}$ pint for women)	150 kcal	225 kcal
3 glasses red wine	300 kcal	
2 glasses red wine		200 kcal
TOTAL	2000 kcal	1400 kcal

Your personal calorie allowance may be higher or lower than 2,000 per day. Turn to pages 20–25 to check yours. Check what your total energy requirement is likely to be by looking at the figure listed alongside your weight in the correct age category and under the heading that most accurately describes your activity level. Knock off

900 calories to create a sufficient deficit to effect a good rate of weight loss. Hopefully, the number of calories you will be burning by taking *additional* exercise will average 200 per day, and this will then create the 1,100 calorie deficit you need each day to achieve a weight loss of approximately 1kg (2lb) per week. Now enter your daily calorie allowance here:

My calorie allowance is _____

Adjust the calories, if necessary, by adding to (or subtracting from) your portion sizes or by adding extra fruit, but do not consume additional alcohol. Women who wish to lose weight on this diet should reduce the portion sizes by approximately 25 per cent unless otherwise stated.

Diet notes
★ 1 piece fresh fruit means 1 average apple, orange etc., or 115g (4oz) any fresh fruit.
★ For guidance, 1 slice regular bread from a large, thin-sliced loaf weighs 25g (1oz). A slice from a large, medium-sliced loaf weighs 40g (1½oz).
★ Unlimited vegetables includes all vegetables, except potatoes, providing they are cooked and served without fat.
★ For sauces and dressings check the nutrition panel on the label before you buy and only select those with 4 grams or less fat per 100 grams of product, except for items such as mustard of which you will consume only minimal amounts.

Breakfasts

Approx. 300 kcal. (Women should reduce portion sizes by 25 per cent.)

★ 1 Low-fat Waffle (see recipe, page 159) served with jam or marmalade.

★ Quick Microwave Porridge with Dried Cherries (see recipe, page 160).

★ Mushroom Frittata (see recipe, page 160) served with unlimited grilled tomatoes and 1 large slice wholemeal toast.

★ Scrambled Eggs with Sun-dried Tomatoes and Smoked Salmon (see recipe, page 161), plus 2 slices wholemeal toast.

★ Potato Hash Browns (see recipe, page 162), plus 2 medium slices wholemeal bread.

★ 1 Toasted Cheese Bagel (see recipe, page 163).

★ 50g (2oz) any cereal with milk (in addition to allowance) and 2 teaspoons sugar, plus 1 piece fresh fruit.

★ 50g (2oz) [dry weight] porridge cooked the night before in water. Serve with milk (in addition to allowance) plus 2 teaspoons sugar or honey.

★ 4 pieces any fresh fruit.

★ 25g (1oz) any cereal with milk (in addition to allowance), and 1 teaspoon sugar, plus 1 medium slice wholemeal toast spread with 2 teaspoons marmalade, honey or preserve.

★ 1 dry-fried or poached egg, 2 St Michael 95% fat-free chipolata sausages, 4 tomatoes, halved and grilled, 115g (4oz) mushrooms cooked in stock (no fat), plus 1 medium slice wholemeal toast.

★ 2 medium slices wholemeal toast topped with 175g (6oz) baked beans and 2 grilled tomatoes.

★ 1 whole grapefruit, 1 poached or boiled egg, and 2 slices wholemeal toast spread with Marmite.

★ 2 bananas plus 200g (7oz) low-fat yogurt, any flavour.

★ Bacon sandwich: 2 rashers lean back bacon, grilled with all fat removed, placed between 2 slices wholemeal bread spread with brown sauce or ketchup or mustard of your choice.

★ 3 Weetabix plus 150ml (¼ pint) milk (in addition to allowance) and 2 teaspoons sugar.

★ 2 Shredded Wheat with 150ml (¼ pint) milk (in addition to allowance) and 2 teaspoons sugar.

★ 3 grilled turkey rashers, 1 slice wholemeal toast topped with 175g (6oz) baked beans, and 2 large, grilled tomatoes.

★ ½ melon, 225g (8oz) grapes, plus 200g (7oz) low-fat yogurt.

★ 2 medium slices wholemeal bread spread with mustard (if liked) plus 75g (3oz) wafer-thin ham.

Lunches

Approx. 450 kcal. (Women should reduce portion sizes by a third.)

★ Coronation Chicken (see recipe, page 164), plus salad with fat-free dressing and 50g (2oz) French bread.

★ Prawn and Pasta Salad (see recipe, page 165), plus 50g (2oz) French bread and 1 piece fresh fruit.

★ Potato and Watercress Salad (see recipe, page 166), plus additional salad with fat-free dressing, 115g (4oz) French bread and 1 piece fresh fruit.

★ Thai Noodle Salad (see recipe, page 165), plus 50g (2oz) French bread and 1 pot low-fat yogurt (max. 100 kcal).

★ Curried Chicken and Yogurt Salad (see recipe, page 167), served with 50g (2oz) French bread and a large green salad with fat-free dressing.

★ Quick Tuna Pâté (see recipe, page 168), served with 50g (2oz) French bread or toast, plus salad with fat-free dressing.

★ Potted Smoked Trout (see recipe, page 168), served with 50g (2oz) French bread and salad with fat-free dressing, plus 1 low-fat yogurt (max. 100 kcal).

★ French Onion Soup (see recipe, page 169), plus 115g (4oz) French bread.

★ Double Soup of Red and Yellow Peppers (see recipe, page 170), plus 50g (2oz) French bread, and 1 low-fat yogurt (max. 100 kcal).

★ Pumpkin and Ginger Soup (see recipe, page 171), plus 115g (4oz) French bread and 1 piece fresh fruit.

★ Chunky Vegetable Soup (see recipe, page 172), plus 115g (4oz) French bread.

★ Caramelised Onion and Lemon Soup with Chive and Parsley Cream (see recipe, page 173), plus 115g (4oz) French bread.

★ Smoked Fish and Corn Chowder (see recipe, page 174), plus 50g (2oz) French bread and 1 piece fresh fruit.

★ Beef Stroganoff (see recipe, page 175), plus 50g (2oz) [dry weight] rice and 1 piece fresh fruit.

★ Smoked Ham Macaroni Cheese (see recipe, page 177), plus 50g (2oz) French bread.

★ The Ultimate BLT (see recipe, page 178) with extra salad, plus 1 low-fat yogurt (max. 100 kcal).

★ Seafood Pancakes with Mustard Sauce (see recipe, page 179), plus salad with fat-free dressing.

★ 1 Italian Toast Topper (see recipe, page 186) served with large salad with fat-free dressing, plus 1 low-fat yogurt (max.100 kcal) and 1 piece fresh fruit.

★ 1 pitta bread filled with salad and topped with either 50g (2oz) wafer-thin ham,chicken,turkey or beef or 75g (3oz) prawns in low-fat dressing.

★ 300ml (½ pint) any soup (max. 4% fat), plus 115g (4oz) chicken with salad in a 50g (2oz) bread roll.

★ 4 slices bread spread with low-fat sauce or dressing and filled with 75g (3oz) wafer-thin ham, beef or chicken and salad, plus 1 banana.

★ Baked Ginger Stuffed Tomatoes (see recipe, page 181), served with 50g (2oz) [dry weight] rice and a large salad with fat-free dressing.

★ Spinach Soufflé (see recipe, page 182), served with 50g (2oz) French bread and salad with fat-free dressing

★ Crunchy Bacon and Spaghetti (see recipe, page 183), plus large salad with fat-free dressing.

★ Tuna and Tarragon Pasta (see recipe, page 184), plus salad with fat-free dressing.

★ Cheesy Stuffed Potato (see recipe, page 185), served with large salad with fat-free dressing.

★ French Bread Pizza (see recipe, page 186), plus salad with fat-free dressing.
★ Club Sandwich (see recipe, page 187), plus 1 piece fresh fruit.

Dinners

Approx. 500 kcal. (Women should reduce portion sizes by 25 per cent.)

Meat and poultry

★ Roast Beef with Yorkshire Pudding, Dry-roast Potatoes and Parsnips (see recipe, page 188), served with unlimited other vegetables.
★ Beef and Pepper Skewers with Teriyaki Sauce (see recipe, page 190), served with 50g (2oz) [dry-weight] rice and salad with fat-free dressing.
★ Steak and Kidney Pie (see recipe, page 191), served with 115g (4oz) potatoes and unlimited other vegetables.
★ 225g (8oz) grilled lean rump steak served with 1 medium-sized jacket potato and unlimited green vegetables.
★ Peppered Steak with Chive and Tarragon Sauce (see recipe, page 192), served with 115g (4oz) new potatoes and unlimited other vegetables.
★ Cottage Pie with Leek and Potato Topping (see recipe, page 193), served with 50g (2oz) French bread and salad with fat-free dressing.
★ Beef and Mushroom Cannelloni (see recipe, page 194) served with 50g (2oz) French bread and salad with fat-free dressing.

★ Spaghetti Bolognese (see recipe, page 196), plus salad with fat-free dressing.

★ Pan-fried Liver with Onions and Balsamic Vinegar (see recipe, page 197), served with 115g (4oz) potatoes and unlimited other vegetables.

★ Lamb Burgers (see recipe, page 198), plus 1 medium-sized jacket potato and unlimited other vegetables.

★ Grilled Marinated Lamb with Caramelised Shallots (see recipe, page 198), served with 115g (4oz) potatoes and unlimited other vegetables.

★ Oriental Pan-cooked Pork (see recipe, page 200), served with 50g (2oz) [dry weight] rice, plus salad with fat-free dressing.

★ Ranchero Pie (see recipe, page 201), plus salad with fat-free dressing.

★ Gammon with Pineapple Rice (see recipe, page 203), plus salad with fat-free dressing.

★ Pork and Apple Burgers in Pitta Bread (see recipe, page 202), served with 100g portion St Michael 95% Fat Free Just Bake Chips, plus salad with fat-free dressing.

★ Gingered Pork with Apricots (see recipe, page 205), served with 50g (2oz) [dry weight] rice and unlimited vegetables, excluding potatoes.

★ Pork and Mango Meatballs with Chilli Sauce (see recipe, page 204), served with 50g (2oz) [dry-weight] rice and a large salad with fat-free dressing.

★ 2 pork chops, grilled with all visible fat removed, served with 175g (6oz) mashed potatoes, unlimited green vegetables and apple sauce.

★ Thai Chicken (see recipe, page 206), served with 50g (2oz) [dry-weight] Jasmine rice and 50g (2oz) French bread.

★ Sticky Ginger Chicken (see recipe, page 208), served with 175g (6oz) new potatoes and salad with fat-free dressing.

★ Tarragon Chicken with Mushroom Sauce (see recipe, page 207), plus 175g (6oz) potatoes and unlimited other vegetables.

★ Chicken Liver Stroganoff (see recipe, page 209), served with 50g (2oz) [dry weight] rice, 50g (2oz) French bread and salad with fat-free dressing

★ Basil Chicken (see recipe, page 210), served with 1 medium-sized jacket potato and salad with fat-free dressing.

★ Chicken Curry (see recipe, page 211), served with 75g (3oz) [dry weight] rice.

★ 225g (8oz) roast chicken served with 225g (8oz) Dry-roast Potatoes (see recipe, page 188) and unlimited green vegetables.

★ Turkey Chilli Pasta (see recipe, page 211), plus salad with fat-free dressing.

★ Lemon Roast Turkey with Cornbread Stuffing and Herb Gravy (see recipe, page 212), served with 175g (6oz) Dry-roast Potatoes (see recipe, page 188) and unlimited other vegetables.

Fish
★ Fisherman's Pie (see recipe, page 214), served with 50g (2oz) French bread and unlimited vegetables, excluding potatoes.

* ★ Smoked Haddock Fish Cakes with Caper Sauce (see recipe, page 215), served with 175g (6oz) potatoes and unlimited other vegetables.
* ★ Pan-fried Tuna with Pepper Noodles (see recipe, page 217), served with 50g (2oz) French bread.
* ★ Spicy King Prawns (see recipe, page 218), served with 50g (2oz) [dry-weight] rice, 50g (2oz) French bread and salad with fat-free dressing.
* ★ Smoked Ham and Prawn Jambalaya (see recipe, page 219), served with 75g (3oz) [dry weight] rice.
* ★ Seafood Kedgeree (see recipe, page 220), served with 50g (2oz) French bread and salad with fat-free dressing.
* ★ Roasted Monkfish Chermoula (see recipe, page 220), served with 1 medium-sized jacket potato and salad with fat-free dressing.
* ★ 175g (6oz) grilled salmon served with 225g (8oz) mashed potatoes and unlimited green vegetables.
* ★ 225g (8oz) white fish cooked in any cook-in sauce (max. 4% fat), served with 75g (3oz) [dry weight] rice, plus unlimited green vegetables.

Vegetarian

* ★ Leek and Sun-dried Tomato Risotto Cakes (see recipe, page 222), served with 225g (8oz) potatoes and salad with fat-free dressing.
* ★ Spicy Chickpea Casserole (see recipe, page 223), plus salad with fat-free dressing.
* ★ Bean and Burgundy Casserole (see recipe, page 224), plus 175g (6oz) potatoes and unlimited other vegetables.

★ Stir-fry Quorn (see recipe, page 225), served with 75g (3oz) [dry-weight] rice.

★ Lentil and Potato Pie (see recipe, page 226), served with 50g (2oz) French bread and a large salad with fat-free dressing.

★ Aduki Bean Pie with Potato and Chive Topping (see recipe, page 227), plus large salad with fat-free dressing.

★ Aubergine Tagine with Roast Garlic (see recipe, page 228), served with 175g (6oz) potatoes, 50g (2oz) French bread and salad with fat-free dressing.

★ Minted Saffron Couscous (see recipe, page 230), served with 115g (4oz) potatoes, 50g (2oz) French bread and salad with fat-free dressing.

★ Vegetarian Loaf (see recipe, page 231), served with 115g (4oz) potatoes, unlimited other vegetables and 50g (2oz) French bread.

★ Butternut Squash and Leek Risotto with Sun-dried Tomatoes (see recipe page 232), served with 50g (2oz) [dry weight] rice and a large salad with fat-free dressing.

★ Aubergine and Ginger Parcels (see recipe, page 233), served with 115g (4oz) potatoes and salad with fat-free dressing.

★ Vegetable Crunch (see recipe, page 234), served with 115g (4oz) potatoes and unlimited other vegetables.

★ Marinated Broccoli and Pepper Stir-fry with Noodles (see recipe, page 236), served with 50g (2oz) French bread and a large salad with fat-free dressing.

★ Fennel and Tomato Pasta (see recipe, page 237), served with 50g (2oz) French bread and salad with fat-free dressing.

★ Tagliatelle with Sun-dried Tomato and Coriander Pesto (see recipe, page 239), plus salad with fat-free dressing.

★ Chilli Pasta Bake (see recipe, page 238), plus salad with fat-free dressing.

Desserts

Approx. 100 kcal. You may also select any dessert from the Bachelor's Diet. (Women should reduce portion sizes by 25 per cent.)

★ Apricot Plum/Date Softie (see recipe, page 240).

★ Orange and Ginger Pashka (see recipe, page 241).

★ Rhubarb and Orange Fool (see recipe, page 243).

★ Crunchy Topped Fruit Fool (see recipe, page 244).

★ Tiramisu (see recipe, page 245).

★ 1 Toffee Yogurt Meringue (see recipe, page 246).

★ Baked Bananas with Raspberries (see recipe, page 246).

★ Baked Egg Custard (see recipe, page 247).

★ Baked Stuffed Apple (see recipe, page 248).

★ Baked Banana (see recipe, page 248).

Treats (men only)

Approx. 200 kcal

★ 1 slice Ginger Marmalade Cake (see recipe, page 249).

★ 1 slice Prune and Almond Cake (see recipe, page 250).

★ 1 slice Carrot and Mango Cake (see recipe, page 251).

★ 1 slice Apple Gateau (see recipe, page 252).

★ 1 slice Spicy Fruit and Apple Cake (see recipe, page 253).
★ 1 slice Bran Loaf (see recipe, page 254).
★ 1 slice Vanilla Swiss Roll with Lemon Curd (see recipe, page 255).
★ 2 St Michael 95% Fat Free Crispie Cakes.
★ 1 × ⅙th serving St Michael 95% Fat Free Strawberry Cheesecake.
★ 1 slice St Michael 95% Fat Free Apricot Flapjacks.
★ 1 slice St Michael 95% Fat Free Orange and Lemon Drizzle Cake.
★ 1 St Michael 95% Fat Free Orange and Chocolate Sponge Cake.
★ 1 × ⅙th serving St Michael 95% Fat Free Orange and Passion Fruit Cake.
★ 4 pieces fresh fruit.
★ ½ St Michael 95% Fat Free Pizza.
★ 300ml (½ pint) soup with 1 medium slice bread.
★ 1 Weetabix plus 150ml (¼ pint) milk and 1 teaspoon sugar.
★ 25g (1oz) Rice Krispies plus 150ml (¼ pint) milk and 1 teaspoon sugar.
★ 2 slices toast spread with 2 teaspoons honey, jam or marmalade.

6

Fit Not Fat

Would you like to lose your excess weight faster, feel fitter, look younger and sleep better – all at the same time? I bet you do. Physical activity – or exercise – will help you accomplish all of these things. There's no downside.

Exercise – what it does and why we need it

Any exercise that makes you out of breath works your heart and lungs harder than normal. This type of exercise is called aerobic and is often described as fat-burning exercise because that is exactly what it does. 'Aerobic' means 'with oxygen', and oxygen is simply a fuel, just like the petrol in your car. When we perform aerobic-type activities, such as walking, jogging, cycling and rowing, we are forced to breathe more deeply, as our lungs demand extra oxygen. The heart pumps more blood around the body, which means that more oxygen is getting to the surface of the skin and the muscles. The oxygen calls on the energy stores in the muscles *and* our fat stores to make the 'fuel' we need for exercise, and that makes us lose weight and inches. It is a win-win situation.

The good news, therefore, is that whenever we burn extra oxygen we will definitely be burning a greater amount of fat as well. The two go hand in hand. That is why endurance athletes are so lean. But for maximum fat burning we don't have to work flat out. Exercising aerobically at a moderate level has been proved to be the most efficient way to burn fat, simply because we can keep going for longer. It is also excellent for all-round fitness because it gives our heart and lungs a workout – and we all know how important these organs are.

DID YOU KNOW THAT IF WE DID JUST 20 MINUTES OF AEROBIC EXERCISE THREE TIMES A WEEK, WE WOULD HALVE OUR CHANCES OF HAVING A HEART ATTACK?

One reason for including exercise in a weight-control programme is to increase the daily *total* calorie expenditure. While it is true that the harder we exercise, the more calories we will burn per minute, it is nevertheless a fact that we are able to keep going for longer if we work at a lower intensity. For instance, an average man walking a mile at a rate of three miles per hour will burn around six calories per minute. It will take him 20 minutes to walk that mile, during which time he will have burnt 120 calories. If he jogged slowly at a rate of five miles per hour, he would burn around 10 calories a minute, and over a distance of a mile the calorie expenditure would be around 120. Running a mile at a seven mile per hour pace, which burns around 16 calories a minute, will burn 128 calories. The key to maximum calorie burning, therefore, is to work at the optimum level within your physical capability. If you can run for 20 minutes, obviously you will burn more fat and calories than if you walked for the same length of time. However, if jogging is beyond your current fitness ability but you can walk easily for, say, 40 minutes, then that is better for you.

Aim to do some continuous aerobic activity, whether it be walking, running or working out at a fitness class or gym for 20–30 minutes, three to five times a week. The aerobic equipment at a gym includes the running machine, stepper, exercise bike, rowing machine and the skiing machine. Always start off slowly, at a gentle pace. After five minutes, increase the intensity a little and maintain that for a further 15–20 minutes (slow down in between if you need to but, if possible, do not stop). Then for the last five minutes, lower the pace to cool down before stopping. Learn the four basic stretches on pages 123–125 and always do these at the end of your activity. This will help prevent aching muscles and help restore your body to normality.

Recent research has now indicated that a combination of aerobic and resistance (strength) exercise is best for long-term weight control. Aerobic exercise burns calories and increases our fitness levels, while resistance training or strength work helps build and maintain lean muscle tissue. It also helps maintain our resting metabolic rate as well as burning some calories.

Strength training

The body is made up of groups of muscles, often in pairs. There are hundreds of muscles all over the body, but here we are only concerned about the ones that determine our physique. While one muscle will cause a part of the body to bend in one direction, it needs another muscle (its partner) to return it to the original position.

To improve the general appearance of the body we need to work certain muscle groups that are situated close to the surface of the skin. These are the muscles that, when toned, give us a firm and well-defined body. Men are most concerned about improving the abdominal area. They also want to have a fair amount of muscle bulk in the upper body, plus strong, powerful legs. To achieve this, it is vital to follow a balanced programme so as not to neglect key areas. For example, you need to perform abdominal exercises regularly, but it is also important to work all the back muscles to complement the abdominal work. Likewise in the legs, the muscle at the front of the thigh, the quadriceps, requires strength training to give power in the legs, but you also need to include adequate work on the hamstrings, the muscle at the back of the thigh.

Going back to abdominals, let me dispel a myth. Many people believe that doing 100 sit-ups a day will reduce a beer belly to a six-pack. If you have a large stomach, it is because you are storing fat there, on top of your muscle, and no amount of 'well, it must be muscle because it's rock hard' will change the fact that it is fat. It is a popular belief that you can turn fat into muscle, but muscle and fat are completely different substances and you can't turn one into the other any more than you can turn a cat into a dog.

If you want to lose that pad of fat that lies around your middle, you need to follow a low-fat, calorie controlled diet, which will force your body to burn some of that fat to make up the shortfall created by the reduced calorie intake, and you need to undertake some regular aerobic exercise that will call upon your fat stores to make fuel for energy. In addition, practising abdominal strengthening exercises will tone up the muscle while you lose the fat. My trial dieters lost an average of 10cm (4in) from their waists in eight weeks. Some men lost as much as 20cm (8in), and the least lost was 2.5cm (1in), and the latter was a guy who didn't do much exercise and drank his alcohol allowance – mostly beer – in two sessions rather than evenly across the week.

To make a muscle stronger and bigger we need to 'work' it. When we 'work' it regularly, it gets shorter, stronger and, particularly in the case of men, bulkier. Every time you lift up a heavy box or do weight-lifting exercises you are 'working' specific muscles. An added benefit is that the more muscle you have, the more calories you burn, since muscle is an energy-hungry tissue.

Stretching is the opposite of strengthening. We need to stretch our muscles to increase our flexibility – for instance to enable us to put on a seatbelt, reach high into a cupboard, change a light bulb or put on our shoes. Stretching also helps release chemicals that collect in the muscles when we have worked them hard, and this helps prevent aches and pains after exercising.

Strengthening exercises also help protect our bones. Although osteoporosis (brittle bone disease) affects considerably more women than men, it is a well-known fact that men and women who take regular exercise have a higher bone density (heavier, stronger bones) than non-exercisers, thereby reducing the likelihood of being affected by this debilitating disease. Exercise that causes the muscles to resist weight has the effect of making them pull across the bones, helping to keep them strong. Weight-bearing exercise such as brisk walking and gentle jogging also helps reduce the risk of osteoporosis and is ideal for strengthening the lower half of the body. Using weights for the upper body, as in the Muscle Training Programme in this chapter, combined with the trunk exercises, will ensure that the rest of the body also has strong, healthy bones. Swimming and cycling, however, are non-weight-bearing and, while they help burn fat and aid general fitness, they will not help prevent osteoporosis.

Reducing stress through exercise

Stress has been defined as 'the rate of wear and tear in the body'. The pace of modern-day living means that many of us lead stressful lifestyles. While not all stress is harmful – indeed we need some degree of stress to stay alert and healthy – the sheer pace and pressures of life can, for many, become intolerable and have a serious effect on mental and physical wellbeing.

Our physiological 'fight or flight' responses that were essential for the survival of our primitive ancestors can be unhealthy in modern-day society. Stress and tension have been associated with heart disease, cancer, strokes, infection, asthma attacks, back pain, chronic fatigue, stomach and bowel disorders, headaches, insomnia, immune system depression (leading to more coughs, colds, flu and sore throats), and the list is still being added to by medical scientists.

When something excites or threatens us, the brain activates the hormonal and nervous systems to stimulate the release of hormones necessary for the body's response to stressful situations. The nervous system activates the release of adrenaline from the adrenal glands, which mobilises energy stores and increases heart rate and blood pressure. We are ready for action!

However, if we have no physical outlet, these natural stress responses can have a harmful effect on our health. For example, adrenaline makes the blood clot faster – an advantage in a fight but a disadvantage in the workplace or home where it can cause a heart attack. Glucose and fats are great energy sources when physical action is required, but they can damage and fur up the arteries if they are left in high quantities in the bloodstream in an uptight sedentary person.

If you are a 'hot reactor' – the sort of person who easily flares up – then this stress response can often be exaggerated. Stress hormones flood out, heart rate and blood pressure soar, glucose and fats pour into the bloodstream and the blood-clotting mechanisms are accelerated. If the 'hot reactor' is forced to regularly stew in their own juices, this sets the scene for major health problems. Prolonged exposure to stress hormones eventually suppresses the immune system and reduces our resistance to illness.

Around 50 years ago, a psychologist called Dr Hans Selye, who pioneered the concept of stress, conducted a fascinating experiment to show the anti-stress benefits of exercise. He subjected 10 rats to a four-week programme of mild electric shocks, flashing lights and loud noises. At the end of the month all the rats had died due to the stress that this had on their health. He then repeated the experiment and had 10 rats walk on a treadmill until they were in good physical condition. Then he subjected them to the same stressful programme of mild electric shocks, etc. At the end of the month, all the rats were alive with no serious effects to their health. Dr Selye concluded that physical fitness helped to 'buffer' the health-destroying effects of stress.

Rather more recently, a group of 36 physically inactive women were randomly assigned into either a walking or sedentary control group. The walking group exercised at a brisk pace for 45 minutes a day, five days a week, for 15 weeks. After six weeks the walkers had not only improved their heart-lung fitness but had also improved their psychological wellbeing scores from an average of 70 (indicating a stress problem) to 81 (positive wellbeing), which was maintained throughout the 15-week study. The sedentary controls remained unchanged at around 70. A study of elderly women (average age 73 years) showed psychological wellbeing scores to be significantly higher amongst those who were regular walkers compared to those who were sedentary.

Regular moderate exercise has been consistently shown to minimise the effects of stress. It is relaxing, it counters the tendency to form blood clots, uses the blood fats for energy, lowers stress hormone levels, reduces muscle tension and helps blood circulate more freely around the body. Studies have shown that a brisk walk is as effective as a tranquilliser in reducing stress and tension – and the benefits last longer. In general, moderate aerobic physical activity such as walking, cycling and swimming seems to be more effective than vigorous, exhaustive activity or resistance exercise in helping reduce stress and tension.

Regular exercise favourably influences the hormones and neurotransmitters associated with depression and feelings of anxiety. Many researchers believe that the feeling of wellbeing that comes during and after exercise is due to mood-altering substances such as serotonin, dopamine, encephalins and endorphins. There has been a special interest recently in endorphins, a morphine-like compound released in the brain which can reduce pain, help normalise blood pressure and may induce a feeling of euphoria and wellbeing. It takes around 20 minutes for these endorphins to have an effect, hence the recommendation to take exercise for at least 20–30 minutes on a regular basis.

There's no doubt that regular exercise makes us feel better and better able to cope with the stresses and strains of daily life. A brisk 20-minute lunchtime walk can work wonders after a stressful morning.

This section on stress was written by Dr Kevin Sykes, Director of the Centre for Exercise and Nutritional Science at University College Chester, and first appeared in Rosemary Conley Diet & Fitness Magazine in 1999.

Where to start

If you think that exercise is not for you, then think again. The benefits you will reap from even a modest amount will far outweigh the effort. This section will help you identify a starting point for exercise and then guide you realistically through a programme which will enable you to increase your fitness gradually.

What are the main benefits?

For the heart and lungs

Maintaining a healthy heart and healthy lungs is the most important reason for taking up an exercise programme. The heart is quite simply a muscle and responds to training in the same way as any other muscle in the body. Make it work harder, and it will become stronger and more efficient. It will improve the circulation of your blood, pumping more blood with every single beat, sending oxygen and nutrients to all the major organs in the body. Your Healthy Heart Programme starts on page 116.

For your shape

Men, quite rightly, are just as concerned about their shape as women are. Men are naturally leaner, have more muscle definition and greater strength than women, but today's lifestyles often make this so difficult to achieve. Men do have an advantage over women, though, when it comes down to muscle work, as they have a greater amount of the predominantly male hormone testosterone, the hormone that helps to build muscle. The exercise programme in this book will build muscle where you need it, such as on the upper body and the legs, and help you streamline those areas that carry too much fat, such as the stomach area, helping you to achieve a masculine shape. See page 126 for your Muscle Training Programme.

For fat burning

The more active we are, the more fat we burn. With most of us doing sedentary jobs it is easy to see why we become fatter. Sitting behind a desk or the wheel of a car for long periods of time and not being sufficiently active in everyday life is a major reason for weight gain. It is therefore important to make time for physical activity when you are not at work. All the sections of this exercise programme will help you to burn fat.

Assessing your current fitness level

Thorough and reliable fitness testing should ideally take place in an exercise physiology laboratory using complex equipment. However, by asking yourself a few key questions and recognising a few facts about your fitness level at the start of an exercise programme you can set realistic goals that you are more likely to adhere to. If you are currently unfit, you need to start at the right level and build up gradually. For example, a failed attempt to run only a short distance might cause you to think that true fitness is so far away that you give up and do nothing. This programme aims to help you overcome this and to begin with your eyes open! For each question, tick just one answer that most accurately describes your activity level, and be honest!

Do you take some form of physical exercise
a at least 3 times a week? ☐
b only occasionally? ☐
c never? ☐

Faced with climbing three flights of stairs, would you
a be able to reach the top in one go without any
  difficulty? ☐
b struggle to the top and be gasping for breath? ☐
c look for a lift or escalator? ☐

Do you walk on average
a more than 3 miles per day? ☐
b between 1 and 3 miles per day? ☐
c less than 1 mile per day? ☐

When you travel to work or go out on errands,
would you
a be capable of running for a bus or train? ☐
b consider walking part of the way? ☐
c try to take public transport or your car as
  close to your destination as possible? ☐

At weekends and in the evenings do you spend
most of your free time
a involved in sporting activities? ☐
b getting on with manual jobs around the house? ☐
c sitting in front of the television or reading? ☐

Now give yourself 5 points for every (a) answer you have
ticked, 3 points for every (b) answer and 0 points for
every (c) answer. Add up your total.

★ If you scored 15–25 points you have a good activity level already. You will be quite fit and able to approach any fitness challenge with confidence. You are already doing a good deal of aerobic activity. Keep this going and the diet will do the rest to reduce your weight.

★ If you scored 6–14 points you are moderately active but could do more to improve your fitness level and this will help your weight-loss programme too. Select a challenge that feels achievable and gradually progress to doing more.

★ If you scored up to 5 points there are lots of things you could do quite easily to improve your currently very low fitness level. You have probably just found yourself in some inactive habits that need shaking off. The amazing thing is that the sooner you start being more active, the better you will feel. You'll be very pleasantly surprised, but do start gently, as too much too soon could be a recipe for disaster.

Start easy

Before starting any exercise programme think hard about what activity or exercise you have done recently. If you have not done very much, then your body will initially object to exercise – but, ultimately, exercise works for everyone! Many people think it is not for them because they believe it is too hard. It is only too hard if you do too much too soon, and then two things happen. Firstly, you are put off doing any more because it hurts and it takes you a long time to recover from it and, secondly, you feel you must be so unfit that achieving real fitness is just too ambitious a goal. Give yourself 12 weeks, and I guarantee you will be in better shape. Give it 12 months, and you will never look back!

Fitting exercise into your life

Starting an exercise programme from scratch and sticking to it means making sweeping changes to how you spend your leisure time. It depends *how much* you want to be in better shape and *how realistic* you are about how long it will take. Look at times in the week when it would be possible to be more active. The Jogging Programme on pages 121–122 takes only 30 minutes of your time, but you do need to select a time when you can be sure you will stick to it. Finding an exercise 'buddy' will considerably increase your chances of doing so because few of us like to let people down, and once an arrangement is made you will follow it through.

Look at the Sample Exercise Planner overleaf to see how you can achieve a balanced programme. Now, plan your own weekly exercise schedule, using the blank version on page 269. Tick the three occasions you are going to set aside 30 minutes for your Healthy Heart Programme. The Muscle Training Programme can be even shorter, taking only an average of 15–20 minutes to cover all the major muscle groups. Try to do this on at least two occasions a week. Go for it!

Sample Exercise Planner

	MONDAY	TUESDAY	WEDNESDAY	THURSDAY	FRIDAY	SATURDAY	SUNDAY
MORNING SESSION							
Healthy Heart Programme 30 mins	☐	☐	☐	✔	☐	☐	☐
LUNCHTIME SESSION							
Healthy Heart Programme 30 mins	✔	☐	☐	☐	☐	☐	☐
Muscle Training Session 15 mins	☐	☐	☐	☐	✔	☐	☐
AFTERNOON SESSION							
Healthy Heart Programme 30 mins	☐	☐	☐	☐	☐	☐	✔
EVENING SESSION							
Muscle Training Session 15 mins	☐	✔	☐	☐	☐	☐	☐

And, finally . . .

If you feel that attending an exercise class would be helpful, I strongly recommend that you join a Rosemary Conley Club as some of my trial dieters did. You will be spoilt to death by a majority attendance of women, but you will be able to do an aerobic fat burning workout, followed by toning exercises, under the supervision of a professional instructor. We do have some male members

FITNESS FACTS

★ To improve and maintain your fitness and help weight management take part in some form of physical activity for about 20 minutes, without a break, at least two to three times a week.

★ Stair climbing is a good test of the heart muscles and the circulation. Use the stairs in preference to a lift or escalator whenever possible. If you avoid climbing stairs you are missing an opportunity to get fit!

★ Brisk walking over a distance of at least one mile per day is an excellent form of aerobic exercise.

★ Many people could increase their fitness by just adding a little more exercise to their daily routine.

★ We are 10 times more likely to continue with a fitness programme if we do something we enjoy, so take up an energetic pastime that you love.

★ Use your spare time fruitfully. Look upon your lawn-mowing, your dog-walking and DIY as a workout – and do more!

in our classes and we would like to have more. The male members that come along really enjoy it and are incredibly effective at shifting their weight, often putting the women to shame!

It is clear that from every angle exercise is a must. If you are physically able to do it then you should. Make it a habit, make it fun and see the results. You'll be so glad you did.

The Healthy Heart Programme

Anything that gets you out of breath, preferably for extended periods of time, is good for the heart. Activities such as swimming, gentle jogging and cycling are excellent and should be built up gradually over a period of time so that you can keep going for longer each time. Short, sharp bursts of activity are not good for the heart and lungs as they put undue stress on the heart, particularly if you are generally out of condition, and they are too exhausting for the lungs. Playing squash, for example, consists of short bursts of intense activity followed by periods of inactivity, and so is not good for the heart. You should be heart and lung fit before you play!

Any physical activity or sport that can be performed without a break for at least 12 minutes is described as aerobic. This is the best type of activity for increasing your general level of fitness and improving the efficiency of your heart, lungs and muscles. Also, because the muscles are not being pushed too hard in aerobic activity and there is sufficient oxygen to meet the demands, you can maximise your fat-burning potential and become leaner as you become fitter.

One of the most useful gadgets I have discovered in recent years is called Caltrac. This is a piece of equipment that measures how many calories you burn through activity. You simply attach it to your belt and programme it with your personal details such as your sex, height, weight and age, and it then cleverly calculates how many calories you burn throughout your daily activities. This enables you to clearly identify those days when you have been more active and therefore achieved more calorie expenditure and heart and lung work! Perhaps the most useful lesson I learnt from wearing my Caltrac was to discover how much activity I had to do to burn an extra 100 calories. This certainly made me much more conscious of the calories I ate! If you would like to buy one of these machines, see the back of this book for mail order details.

Walking

Walking is a form of aerobic exercise that everyone can incorporate into their daily routine without too much effort. With every passing decade people have needed to walk less and less each day, due in part to our sedentary lifestyles and our reliance on the car. However, if you change the way you think about walking, particularly because you now know it helps you to burn fat and keeps you healthy, you can find lots of opportunities in the working day to increase the amount of walking you do, for instance by avoiding the lift when the stairs are right next to it or by parking the car further away from the entrance to the office. You could even have two days a week when you leave the car at home and find ways of getting to work that involve walking for part of the journey, for instance by getting off the bus a couple of stops earlier. Try it! No need to put on any kit or set a special time aside, it is the 'anywhere, any time' type of exercise that can make a major contribution to your fitness and fat burning.

Swimming

Swimming can also make a major contribution to your heart and lung efficiency. It uses muscles throughout the whole body and is truly aerobic, ensuring a high level of fat-burning. Gradually decrease the frequency with which you stop to get your breath back and aim to swim continuously at a steady pace for 20 minutes.

Cycling

If you used to enjoy cycling when you were young, the chances are you would easily enjoy it as an adult. Make the commitment of buying a bike and get out on the open road to improve your aerobic fitness. The advantage of cyling over walking and jogging is that you can cover greater distances in a relatively short space of time. And if you can get out into the countryside you have the added benefits of fresh air and scenery. One word of advice: if you do take up cycling, treat yourself to some padded cycle shorts, as these make cycling long distances more comfortable. Take a water bottle to sip from, too. Dehydration is one of the key factors in causing fatigue, so keep hydrated during cycling or, indeed, any form of aerobic exercise.

The development of the National Cycle Network in the UK means that you will be able to cycle safely away from traffic, pollution and noise. This 8,000 mile network will be made up of traffic-free routes. For more information, contact Sustrans, PO Box 21, Bristol, BS99 2HA. (tel. 0117 929 0888 or Website www.sustrans.org.uk).

Another option is to do a charity bike ride. It gives you a goal, encourages you to train and does a load of good for the charity too. In 1998 my husband Mike and three of his friends decided to join the Paris to Lourdes Cycle Ride in aid of three charities. Having a goal to aim for gave these late-thirties, not-as-fit-as they-used-to-be men a reason for getting fit. The 700-mile journey was to be made in just seven days. A tall order by anyone's standards.

I was enlisted to give advice and direction on how they should train and what to eat. Our fortnightly training sessions cum supper parties were great fun. An air of excitement began to fill the atmosphere as the training continued. Richard, James, Chris and Mike became leaner and fitter than they had been for years. They were in great shape as the day approached for their departure in a tiny plane to Paris. They raised a staggering £46,000 between them as well as pushing themselves to their physical limits. Cycling has now become an additional physical activity in their repertoire, alongside golf, horse-riding and squash. Doing the charity bike ride forced them to buy the right kit, train and gave them a real sense of accomplishment. Unless Mike has a challenge like that he is not sufficiently motivated to make the effort. If you are like that, look for a physical challenge that will motivate you!

If you decide to do a charity bike ride, build up your distances gradually and keep a record of the miles you achieve. After each ride do the stretches on pages 123–125. These are very important as they will help you avoid discomfort later. Also do some strength exercises (see the Muscle Training Programme on page 126). These will have the effect of making your muscles bigger and more powerful so that they are able to do more work. Take a rest day after every third day of training to allow the muscles to recover so that you avoid injury.

Jogging

Anyone who has tried jogging will tell you how hard it is, but it is one of the most effective ways of developing excellent heart and lung fitness and controlling weight. The pressure on the joints can be a problem and you should build up through a walking phase first to reduce the risk of injury. If you have a bad back or are very over-weight at the start of the programme, proceed with caution. Follow the Back Conditioning Programme (see page 144) to help you strengthen some key areas.

Most people who start a jogging programme try to do too much too soon, making it impossible to sustain. The Jogging Programme that follows is different because it shows you how to build up gradually. If you are determined to stick to it, you will succeed. To help keep you motivated, consider investing in a Caltrac (see page 116) and use it consistently over the period of time that you build up your jogging. You will then see the amazing effect that the programme has on your calorie expenditure and, consequently, your ability to lose weight.

The programme recommends starting with a walking phase. Continuous walking will slowly prepare your legs for the next jogging phase and will also help you to develop a consistent routine. The programme always takes exactly 30 minutes and you are advised to do it no more than three times a week. It builds from exclusively walking to only jogging over a period of 12 weeks. Once you can run for 30 minutes, three times a week, you will be doing all that you need to for heart and lung fitness. To tone your muscles, simply add the Muscle Training Programme on the other days of the week.

I must stress, however, that jogging does not suit everyone. If you hate jogging, do something else – go cycling or swimming instead. The best exercise for you is the one that you enjoy and that you do regularly.

Jogging Programme

If you have never walked at a brisk pace continuously for 30 minutes you may need to build up slowly. Start by trying to fit shorter bouts of walking into your normal day (even 10 minutes is a start) until you can comfortably keep going briskly for 30 minutes.

Follow the programme on just three days a week. Place a tick under columns 1, 2 and 3 as you complete each challenge. Always finish each session by doing the stretches at the end of this section.

	DAY 1	DAY 2	DAY 3
WEEK 1 Walk 30 minutes	☐	☐	☐
WEEK 2 Walk 30 minutes	☐	☐	☐
WEEK 3 Jog 2 minutes, walk 4 minutes Complete sequence 5 times	☐	☐	☐
WEEK 4 Jog 3 minutes, walk 3 minutes Complete sequence 5 times	☐	☐	☐

	DAY 1	DAY 2	DAY 3

WEEK 5
Jog 5 minutes, walk 2½ minutes
Complete sequence 4 times

☐ ☐ ☐

WEEK 6
Jog 7 minutes, walk 3 minutes
Complete sequence 3 times

☐ ☐ ☐

WEEK 7
Jog 8 minutes, walk 2 minutes
Complete sequence 3 times

☐ ☐ ☐

WEEK 8
Jog 9 minutes, walk 2 minutes
Complete sequence twice and
then run for 8 minutes

☐ ☐ ☐

WEEK 9
Jog 9 minutes, walk 1 minute
Complete sequence 3 times

☐ ☐ ☐

WEEK 10
Jog 13 minutes, walk 2 minutes
Complete sequence twice

☐ ☐ ☐

WEEK 11
Jog 14 minutes, walk 1 minute
Complete the sequence twice

☐ ☐ ☐

WEEK 12
Jog 30 minutes

☐ ☐ ☐

Standing Stretch Programme

Do these stretches after completing any activity from the Healthy Heart Programme. Stretching is a vital part of the cooling-down process and allows the muscles to return to their original length after the continuous shortening that occurs whenever we do repetitive work on them. It also allows the muscle fibres to be pulled apart, allowing more blood to flow through the muscle, which helps prevent muscle soreness. Stretching also helps promote and maintain elasticity in the muscles, thereby keeping you supple and flexible. The regular exerciser who does not stretch is far more likely to suffer injury, because the muscles become tight and inflexible.

Calf stretch

Begin facing a wall with one leg behind the other. Keeping the back leg straight, bend the front leg. Place your hands on the wall for support and lean forward into the front leg to feel a stretch in the calf of the back leg. Make sure both feet point straight ahead and take the back leg further back to feel more of a stretch. Hold for 8 seconds, then release. Change legs and repeat.

Hamstring stretch

Take one leg up on to a surface that is hip height (a stool or work surface is ideal). Keeping the other leg straight, lean forwards, moving from the hip rather than the spine, and feel a strong stretch at the back of the thigh of the raised leg. Hold for 10 seconds, then lean forward more and hold for a further 10 seconds. Change legs and repeat.

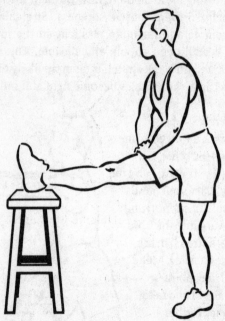

Quadricep stretch

Place one hand on a wall for support, bend the opposite leg up behind you and grip the ankle. Keep the knee of the standing leg slightly bent and push the hip of the other leg forward to feel a stretch down the front of the

thigh. Hold for 8 seconds,
then change legs and repeat.

Inner thigh stretch

Place your left foot on
the seat of a chair with
the toe pointing
forward and the knee
of the standing leg
slightly bent.
Now bend your
trunk towards the
right leg to feel a
stretch in the inner
thigh of the
raised leg.

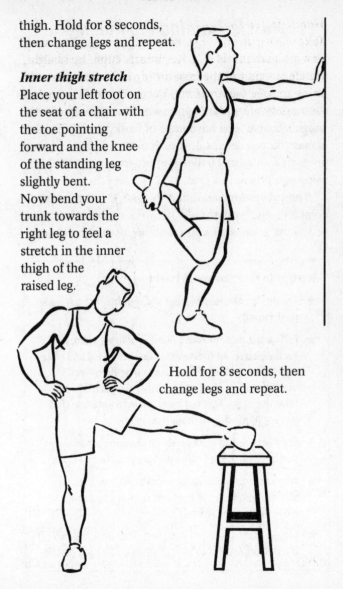

Hold for 8 seconds, then
change legs and repeat.

Muscle Training Programme

This programme is a good introduction to building muscle strength in the comfort of your own home, targeting exactly the areas you need to tone. It is a great starter programme for anyone who has not worked with weights before. The advantage of working with weights is that you can see results much more quickly and then progress to a more challenging programme, perhaps by using equipment in a gym.

The programme should only take 15–20 minutes to complete and you should perform it on at least two occasions a week. If you combine it with the Healthy

---

Top tips to effective weight training

★ Try all the exercises without the weights first to check positioning.

★ Follow the recommended number of repetitions for each exercise. As soon as that feels too easy add more repetitions to the point where you begin to feel uncomfortable, then add a further 4 repetitions to fully 'overload'. This is a good guide to ensuring that you are improving without risking injury.

★ Start with only a moderately challenging set of dumbbells – 3.5kg (7lb) – and progress to 5kg (10lb).

★ When using dumbbells, always keep the wrists in a straight line with the forearms so that you avoid movement in the wrists.

★ Always warm up before you start. Step up and down off the bottom step of a flight of stairs and/or jog on the

---

Heart Programme, you will then be taking exercise on five occasions a week, but the total time spent exercising will only be two hours per week! Of course you could do more, and you probably will when it becomes a way of life, but by exercising for just two hours a week, you will soon see significant changes in your body shape and greatly improve the strength of your heart and lungs. You will feel like a new man!

When people first undertake a muscle training programme they usually do too much too soon and end up very sore. This is because when we put demands on our muscles there is a point at which they are comfortable, then a point at which they are 'overloaded', and finally a

---

spot for a minimum of 5 minutes, and simulate some of the moves without weights first.

★ It is important to isolate the muscle area being worked by 'fixing' the rest of the body. If you don't keep the rest of the body static, you will reduce the amount of work the muscle does and risk injury.

★ Always breathe out on the effort, usually through the lifting phase of the exercise.

★ If you are sore, you are simply doing too much. Reduce the number of repetitions and build up more gradually.

★ Always stretch before and after your programme. Follow the stretches at the end of this section.

★ Be consistent. Decide how many times a week you are going to do the programme – 2–3 times is the recommendation – and then stick to it! You will not get results unless you adhere to it.

point at which they are 'overworked'. It is the overworked phase that is the most damaging, and if you are new to exercise you should make sure that you take each muscle only to the point of 'overload', where you begin to feel you are working hard but definitely not reaching a burning sensation. A burning sensation indicates that you are beginning to build up lactic acid in the muscle, and too much lactic acid damages muscle tissue, leading to a build-up of scar tissue.

Upper body exercises

Biceps curl

Stand with feet apart, holding a dumbbell in each hand, and have your arms close by your sides. Now, keeping the elbows close to the waist, bend the forearms up towards the shoulders. Lower under control. Repeat 10 times, then rest and repeat.

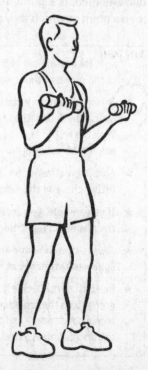

Upright row

Begin with both
dumbbells held in front
of the body and the backs
of your hands facing forward.
Keep your shoulders back and
your head up as you lift the
weights up towards the chin,
bringing the elbows higher than
the shoulders. Lower under
control. Repeat 8 times, then
rest and repeat.

Lat pulls

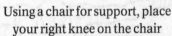

Using a chair for support, place
your right knee on the chair
and hold the back of the
chair with your right
hand. Hold one dumbbell
in the left hand, lean
forward slightly and
raise the bent elbow
up behind you as far
as possible without
twisting the trunk,
then lower it again. Do 10
repetitions, then change
arms and repeat.

Triceps extension
Using the chair as
in the previous
exercise, start with
the elbow up behind.
From there, extend the arm
until just before the elbow locks
out, then slowly release.
Repeat 8 times, then change
arms and repeat.

Deltoid raise
Stand with feet apart and
hold a dumbbell in each
hand. Keeping the
elbows slightly

bent, lift both arms out
to the sides to just
above shoulder height
and lower them
again. Keep the rest
of the body static.
Breathe out as you
lift and in as you
lower. Do 8
repetitions, then
rest and repeat.

Overhead press

Begin with the weights on your shoulders. Now, under control, push the weights overhead until they almost meet, then lower them slowly. Repeat 6 times, then rest and repeat.

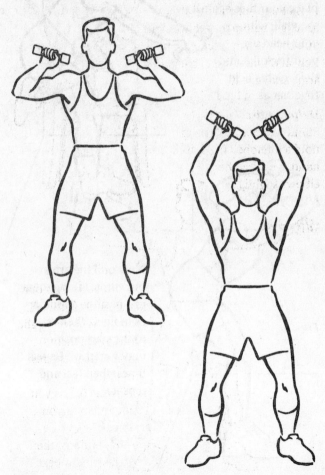

Prone flyes

Hold a dumbbell in each hand and stand about 60cm (2ft) from a wall. Now lean forward and place your hips against the wall, with your head up, your back flat and the weights held together as in fig. 1.

Fig. 1

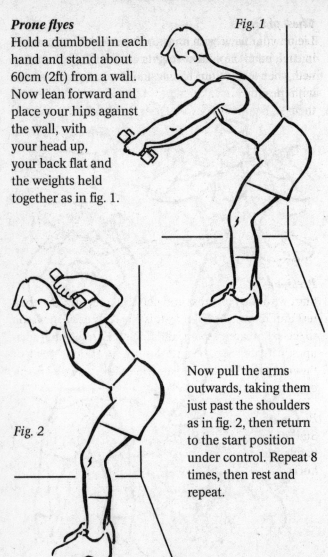

Now pull the arms outwards, taking them just past the shoulders as in fig. 2, then return to the start position under control. Repeat 8 times, then rest and repeat.

Fig. 2

Chest press

Lie on your back with knees bent and hold a dumbbell in each hand. Hold the weights close to your shoulders with your elbows out to the side. Now, forming an arc with the weights, take them above the chest, and lower them again under control. Do 8, then rest and repeat.

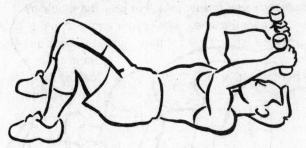

Press-up

Start with the box press and perform 8 repetitions, then rest and repeat. As soon as this feels too easy, move on to the extended press-up, and finally on to the full press-up, still aiming to perform 2 sets of 8 repetitions. In all of the press-up exercises, breathe in on the way down and out on the way up

Box press
Start on your
hands and
knees,

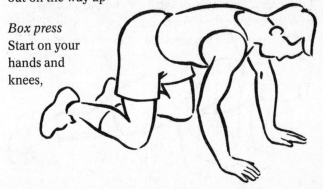

with your wrists underneath the shoulders, your abdominals pulled in and your back flat. Lower your forehead to the floor, then push back up again, without locking the elbows.

Extended press-up
Place the knees further back, but keep the shoulders over the wrists. Lower your forehead to the floor, then push back up again, without locking the elbows.

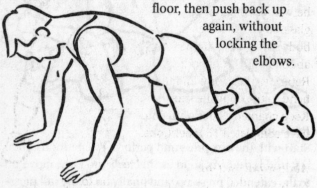

Full press-up
Extend the legs fully, with the knees off the floor. Lower the chest towards the floor and push up again, without locking the elbows. Take care not to arch the spine, and keep your abdominals pulled in tight and your back flat.

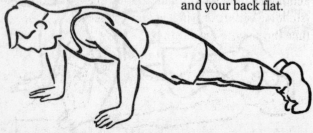

Trunk exercises

Lateral side bends

Stand with feet apart and hold
a dumbbell in each hand.
Now bend to one side
without leaning forward or
back, as if moving
between two panes of
glass. Keep the lower
body still, pulling in the
abdominals throughout.
Return to the centre and then
bend to the opposite side.
Keep changing sides until you
have completed 16 repetitions.

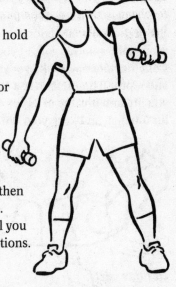

Abdominal pull-ins

Lie on your back with knees bent and feet flat on the
floor. Breathe in and, at the same time, push your ribs
and stomach area outwards. As you breathe out pull
them in and flatten them against the spine. Hold for 4
seconds, then release and repeat 4 times altogether.
This exercise really helps you to focus on your
abdominal muscles and can be done in any position
(standing, sitting or lying) at any
time throughout the day.

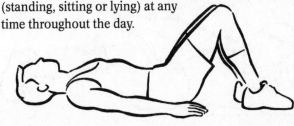

Abdominal curls

Lie on your back with knees bent and feet flat on the floor. Place both hands behind your head to support the neck. Pull your abdominals in and flatten them against the spine as you lift your head and shoulders from the floor and look over your knees. Lower again and repeat 8 times, then rest and repeat. Breathe out as you lift, and breathe in as you lower. Do not attempt to lift too high and keep your chin off your chest.

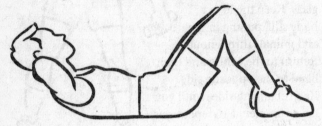

Oblique curls

Lie on your back with knees bent and feet flat on the floor. Place your right hand behind your head and your left hand on the right thigh. Slide the hand up the leg as you lift your head and shoulders off the floor, so that the trunk twists slightly towards the right. Lower slowly and repeat 8 times on one side. Change sides and repeat.

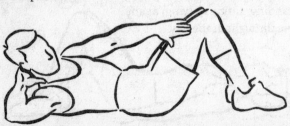

Reverse curls

Lie on your back with the feet off the floor, knees bent and feet together. The thighs should be at a right angle to the hips. Keep your arms by your sides and perform the abdominal pull-ins as before as you breathe out and lift the knees slightly towards the ceiling. Repeat 6 times, then rest and repeat.

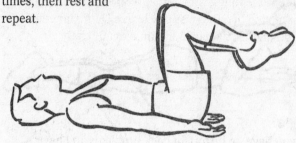

Back raises

Lie on your front and, depending on the condition of your back, choose one of these three positions.

Fig. 1

If you have a bad back, keep your forearms on the floor in front of you and lift the upper body from the floor. Keep looking at the floor so that the neck remains in a neutral position. Lower slowly and repeat 6 times. Breathe out as you lift and breathe in as you lower.

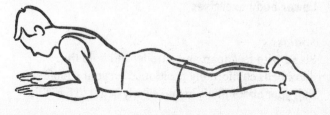

Fig. 2

If you do not have a bad back but feel you have a weak back, place the elbows close to the waist and have the palms facing up. Keep looking at the floor as you slowly lift the upper body, then lower it again under control. Repeat 6 times, then rest and repeat.

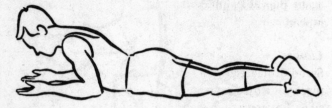

Fig. 3

If you have no history of back problems and have exercised previously, place your arms by your sides and slowly lift the upper body from the floor, then lower again under control. Repeat 6 times, then rest and repeat.

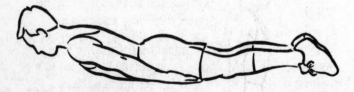

Lower body exercises

Squats

Stand with feet apart and parallel and hold the dumbbells comfortably positioned on your shoulders. Pull your abdominals in and slowly begin to bend the

knees, pushing your hips back and
keeping the knees in line with
the toes. Keep looking
forwards and keep
your back straight as
you bend. Slowly lift up
again. Repeat 10 times, then rest
and repeat.

Lunges

Stand with feet together and
place your arms at your
sides, holding a dumbbell
in each hand. Now take a
large step forward with the
right leg, making sure

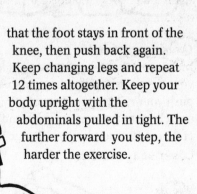

that the foot stays in front of the
knee, then push back again.
Keep changing legs and repeat
12 times altogether. Keep your
body upright with the
abdominals pulled in tight. The
further forward you step, the
harder the exercise.

Muscle Training Stretch Programme

Hamstring stretch

Sit with your right leg straight and your left leg comfortably bent in front of you. Place both hands to either side of your right knee and, keeping your back straight, lean forward slightly until you feel a stretch in the back of the thigh of the right leg. Hold for 10 seconds, then lean forward further and hold for another 10 seconds. Change legs and repeat.

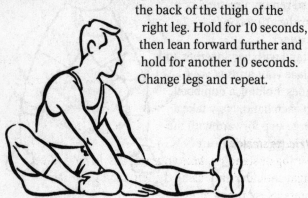

Quadriceps stretch

Lie on your front, bend your right leg and take hold of your right ankle. Keep the right knee on the floor but push your right hip further into the floor to feel a stretch in the front of the thigh and up into the hip. Hold for 10 seconds, then change legs and repeat.

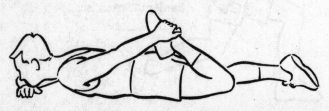

Inner thigh stretch

Sit on the floor and place the soles of your feet together. Hold your ankles and press down on your knees to push them further towards the floor. Keep your head up and your back straight. Hold for 10 seconds, then apply more pressure for a further 10 seconds.

Triceps stretch

Sitting or standing, take your right hand behind your right shoulder and, using the left hand to apply pressure on the right underarm, push the right arm further behind you so that it moves further down your back. Keep your back straight and keep looking forward. Hold for 8 seconds, then change arms and repeat.

Deltoid stretch

Take your right arm across in front of your body, keeping it straight. Use your left hand to apply pressure to push the right arm further across to feel a stretch at the back of the right shoulder. Hold for 8 seconds, then change arms and repeat.

Pectoral stretch

Sitting or standing, take both arms behind your back and clasp your hands. Keep the elbows bent as you pull your shoulder blades together to feel a stretch across the chest. Hold for 8 seconds, then release.

Trapezius stretch

Sitting or standing, take both arms out in front of you at shoulder height, with your head down. Now round your spine and extend the arms further away from the shoulders to feel a stretch across the back of the shoulders. Hold for 8 seconds, then release.

Abdominal stretch

Lie on your front with your forearms placed comfortably in front of you. Now lift your upper body from the floor, keeping your elbows on the floor. Pull your chin forward slightly and feel a stretch in the front of the trunk. Hold for 8 seconds, then release.

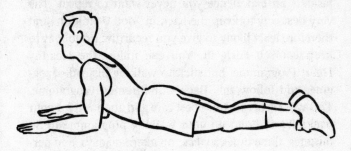

Spine stretch

Come up onto your hands and knees, and slowly pull in the abdominals, arching your back up at the same time. Tuck the head and hips under as far as possible and hold for 6 seconds, then release. Breathe normally throughout.

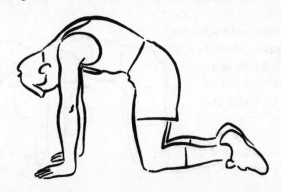

Back Conditioning Programme

Back problems are a major concern and have a considerable effect on our lives. Suddenly finding yourself unable to move because your back has seized up and not being able to perform even the most basic of daily tasks is an experience you never want to repeat. The very best way to keep the back in good condition, and therefore least likely to give you recurring trouble, is to keep yourself fairly fit. You can follow the Healthy Heart Programme, but stick to walking instead of jogging, and follow this Back Conditioning Programme. This will ensure the very best care and attention for your back. Try to build up your walking programme to 30 minutes, three times a week, on alternate days, and perform the conditioning exercises on the days in between. If any of the exercises feel uncomfortable, avoid them and stick with those that suit. A bad back takes many forms and you may have to work at finding the exercises that work for you. Generally speaking, you need to concentrate on the abdominal exercises as these are most likely to give you real help.

Abdominal hollowing
Position yourself on
your hands and
knees, with your
hands under the

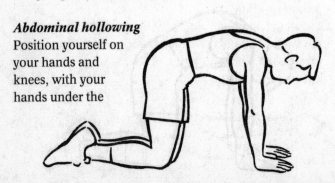

shoulders and your knees under the hips. Allow the stomach area to sag down, then pull it tight and up as if trying to touch your tummy button to your spine. Try not to move your spine and hips. Hold for 6 seconds, then release. Perform 4 times altogether.

Easy abdominal curls
Lie on your back with your knees bent and feet flat on the floor, hip distance apart. Place your right hand behind your head and your left hand on top of your left thigh. Now, keeping your chin off your chest, slowly lift the head and shoulders off the floor, sliding the hand further up towards the knee, then release back down again. Breathe out as you lift and breathe in as you lower. Repeat 6 times, then rest and repeat.

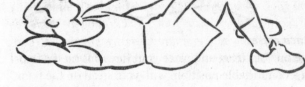

Spinal rotation
Lie on the floor with your right arm out in a 'T' position. Bend the right knee and rotate the trunk towards the left leg, bringing the right knee towards the floor

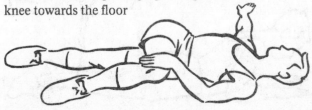

and using your left hand to press the right knee to the floor. Try to keep the right shoulder on the floor. Hold for 6 seconds, then slowly release and repeat to the other side.

Spinal mobility

Position yourself on your hands and knees. Pull the abdominal area in tight and, at the same time, pull your spine up towards the ceiling, tucking the head and hips under as far as possible. Lower slowly to the starting position. Repeat slowly and rhythmically 4 times altogether.

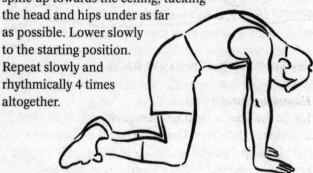

Back raises

Lie on your front and place your forearms on the floor in a comfortable position, with your head on the floor. Keep your head looking down at the floor and slowly lift the upper body, keeping the elbows on the floor throughout. Slowly lower again and repeat 6 times altogether.

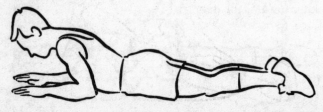

Superman extensions

Lie on your front with your arms extended on the floor in front of you. Now slowly lift the right arm and the left leg at the same time, then lower them again. Repeat with the left arm and right leg. Keep changing arms and legs until you have completed 8 repetitions.

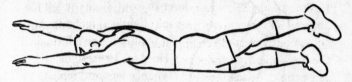

Key Stretches that Help Bad Backs

Hamstring stretch

Lie on the floor with knees bent. Bring the right knee and hip to 90 degrees. Grip your hands behind the right knee and straighten the leg to feel a stretch at the back of the thigh. The knee should remain directly above the hip.

Hold for 10 seconds, then rest. Repeat with the other leg.

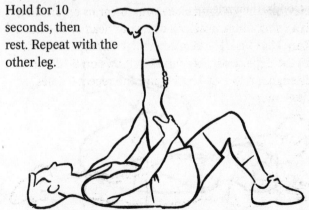

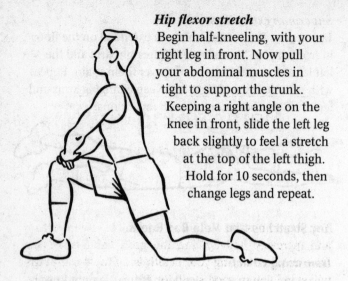

Hip flexor stretch

Begin half-kneeling, with your right leg in front. Now pull your abdominal muscles in tight to support the trunk. Keeping a right angle on the knee in front, slide the left leg back slightly to feel a stretch at the top of the left thigh. Hold for 10 seconds, then change legs and repeat.

Lower back stretch

Lie on the floor and bring your knees up towards your chest. Grip behind the thighs, bringing your knees into your chest and up towards your shoulders. Hold for 10 seconds, then release.

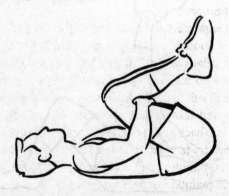

7

Maintaining Your New Weight

You should now be well into the swing of low-fat eating and increased activity, and the good habits that you have acquired during your health and fitness campaign will stand you in good stead for life. So, once you have reached your desired weight, don't go back to your old, bad habits. Eating healthily and keeping active will pay enormous dividends, not just in terms of your weight and your body shape but also in terms of your overall health and wellbeing. You've done the tough bit; now hold on to that progress.

You can now relax the rules a little and increase the quantities of food you eat. You may add a few more dressings to salads and eat a little low-fat hard cheese, but if you are to maintain your new figure and energy levels you will still need to follow a predominantly low-fat formula and take regular exercise. We only regain weight if we go back to our old, bad habits. So, continue to eat low fat, try to exercise at least three times a week for at least 20 minutes each time, and you should have no trouble in maintainng your progress.

The good news is that after a few weeks on a low-fat eating regime, your tastebuds adapt – for many the taste of fatty foods becomes repulsive – and so it should be relatively simple to stick with your new low-fat way of eating and keep the excess weight off for good. But, if you start eating butter and cheese again, you'll be astounded at how quickly you'll fall back to your old habits and regain the weight. And, once you are used to a regular programme of activity, you will feel so good that, hopefully, you will want to keep it up, but if you do stop it will be difficult to find the discipline to get going again!

Keep an eye on the scales and the fit of your trousers. If you find you are gaining weight again, return to the diet or cut back on the quantities you are eating. If you take immediate action, you can remedy any damage quite swiftly.

If you dine out regularly, select carefully from the menu. By all means eat the bread roll, but refrain from putting butter or margarine on it. Choose a light starter such as melon or a vegetable-based soup. For your main course, choose a fish or chicken dish that isn't deep-fried and ask for vegetables to be served without butter. Select a fruit-based dessert or a sorbet (pavlova is also fine if you have the willpower to leave the cream!) and try to avoid the cheese board. If you can't resist, just have a small portion of your favourite cheese. Drink still or sparkling mineral water alongside your wine as this will help fill you up. But most of all, enjoy it! If you only eat out occasionally and your regular food is predominantly low in fat, you can be less strict on these special occasions.

Remember, eating should be a pleasurable experience, and by following the advice you have read in this book you should still be able to eat well and heartily and feel better for it.

Ten tips for weight maintenance

1 Eat three meals a day and eat low-fat, high-volume foods. Not only will these fill you up, they will cause your body to work harder and burn more calories during the digestion process.

2 Remember that the fat you eat becomes fat on your body. If you want to stay lean you have to eat lean. Use the lists on the following pages for a quick and easy check on which foods to eat and which to avoid.

3 Do not eat between meals. Nibbling between meals can seriously damage your waistline.

4 Avoid temptation by not keeping biscuits and sweets in easy reach. Instead, have plenty of fresh fruit available and keep the refrigerator stocked with low-calorie drinks and low-fat yogurts to satisfy sweet cravings.

5 Don't skip meals, since this can lead to uncontrolled eating later, and always eat breakfast to help kick-start your metabolism each day.

6 The occasional indiscretion is not the end of the world, but do remember that one lapse can lead to another, so indulge with caution! Don't let a minor lapse become a major relapse.

7 Continue to be as physically active as possible. Aerobic exercise will keep your heart fitter, will burn fat and also keep your metabolic rate buoyant so that weight maintenance becomes easier.

8 Exercise should always be enjoyable. Try to vary your activities so that you don't get bored.

9 Practise good posture habits at all times throughout the day. Good posture habits will keep you looking more youthful.

10 Remember that *you* are in control of your body and your lifestyle. If you want to stay slim and fit, you *can* do it.

Making the right food choices

The following lists itemise foods that form the basis of a healthy diet which will enable you to maintain your new lower weight and foods which should only be eaten occasionally or avoided altogether if possible. You may select freely from List 1 without worrying about quantities unless it specifies 'in moderation'. You may also select occasionally from List 2, but try to avoid items from List 3.

LIST 1
Most of the following foods may be eaten freely, but restrict the quantities of those specified to be consumed in moderation.

Alcohol: do not exceed 28 units a week for men and 21 units a week for women.
Beans, lentils and pulses: any type.
Bread: any type without added fat (i.e. not fried, no butter or margarine).
Breakfast cereal: any type.
Cakes: cakes made with little or no fat.
Cheese: cottage cheese, fromage frais, quark.

Condiments: (see also *Sauces*.) any type.

Crispbreads: rye crispbreads, Ryvita or other low-fat brands.

Dressings: lemon juice, oil-free dressings, vinegar, any dressings with a maximum of 4% fat. Reduced-oil dressings in moderation.

Eggs: egg whites can be eaten freely. Limit whole eggs to 3 a week.

Fish (including shellfish): any type, e.g. cod, plaice, halibut, whiting, lemon sole, cockles, crab, lobster, mussels, oysters, prawns, salmon, shrimps, tuna in brine, mackerel, herrings, kippers, sardines in tomato sauce, rollmop herrings, sprats – all cooked without butter and not fried.

Flour: any type.

Fruit: any type of fresh, frozen or tinned fruit, except avocado, coconut and olives. Dried fruit in moderation.

Fruit juices: apple juice, exotic fruit juices, grapefruit, grape juice, unsweetened orange and pineapple.

Game: any type, roasted, without fat and with all skin removed.

Grains: any type.

Gravy: made with gravy powder or low-fat granules (max. 4% fat).

Jams, preserves and spreads: honey, jam, Marmite, Bovril, marmalade, syrup – all in moderation.

Meat: any lean red meat cooked without fat, low-fat sausages (max. 4% fat), e.g. St Michael Extra Lean Pork Sausages.

Meat substitutes: textured vegetable protein (TVP), Quorn, vegeburgers, soya.

Milk: skimmed or semi-skimmed.

Nuts: chestnuts only.

Offal: any type cooked without fat.

Pasta: any type served without fat.

Pickles and relishes: any type.

Pizza: any type with 4% or less fat.

Poultry: chicken, duck, turkey – all cooked without fat and with all skin removed.

Prepared meals: any range with 4% or less fat.

Puddings: custard (made with skimmed milk), fresh fruit salad, low-fat fromage frais, fruit cooked with wine, jelly, meringues, rice pudding made with skimmed milk, low-fat yogurt, pavlova made with yogurt, any ready-made pudding with 4% or less fat.

Rice: brown or white, boiled or steamed.

Sauces: apple, brown, cranberry, horseradish, mint, tomato ketchup, soy sauce, low-fat white sauces, Worcestershire, tartare.

Snacks: any type with 4% or less fat.

Soups: any with 4% or less fat.

Soya

Stuffing: made with water.

Sugar: any type in moderation, artificial sweeteners.

Vegetables: any type (except ackee and avocado) cooked and served without fat.

Yogurt: any low-fat varieties.

LIST 2

You may occasionally select items from this list.

Bread: bread spread with low-fat spreads.

Cakes and biscuits: Jaffa Cakes, filo pastry, savoury biscuits such as cream crackers and water biscuits.

Cheese: cheese spread, Edam, Gouda, low-fat hard cheese, low-fat soft cheese.

Confectionery: any fat-free types.

Dressings: low-fat mayonnaise.

Drinks: low-fat malted drinks such as low-fat brands of Horlicks, Ovaltine, drinking chocolate – all made with skimmed milk. Tea and coffee with skimmed or semi-skimmed milk, yogurt drinks.

Egg and egg products: all types in moderation. Yorkshire pudding made with skimmed milk and cooked in a non-stick baking tin without fat.

Fats and spreads: low-fat spreads with less than 10% fat.

Fish: fish fingers (grilled), fish in sauces (branded products).

Jams and preserves: lemon curd in moderation.

Meat and meat products: beef burgers (grilled), corned beef, faggots, lamb chops (grilled), low-fat sausages (grilled), meat with some fat such as streaky bacon, roast meat.

Milk, cream and similar products: Dream Topping, full-fat milk, single cream.

Puddings: regular custard, ice-cream (except Cornish varieties), pavlova, regular rice pudding, sponge flans, trifle.

Sauces: sweet and savoury sauces made with full-fat milk (no butter), e.g. parsley sauce, white sauce.

Soups: any soup.

Sugar: syrup.

Take-away meals: ask for those cooked with minimal or little fat.

Vegetables: thick-cut chips, oven chips.

Yogurt: creamy yogurts, Greek yogurt.

LIST 3
Avoid the following foods whenever possible.

Bread: garlic bread.

Cakes and biscuits: all cakes and pastries not included in Lists 1 and 2, all sweet biscuits, savoury biscuits containing cheese or butter.

Cheese: full-fat cheeses of any kind.

Confectionery: butterscotch, caramel, chocolate, fudge, toffees.

Dressings: all oils, cream dressings, French dressings, regular mayonnaise.

Drinks: cocoa and cocoa products, e.g. Ovaltine, except low-fat varieties, regular Horlicks, tea or coffee with cream.

Eggs and egg products: custard tarts, egg custards, quiches, Scotch eggs, Yorkshire pudding cooked in fat.

Fats and spreads: butter, dripping, lard, low-fat spreads with more than 50% fat content, margarine, margarines high in polyunsaturates, oil (all kinds), peanut butter, suet.

Fish: fish in batter, fried fish, fried fish cakes, kippers in butter, fried whitebait.

Fruit: avocado pears.

Meat and meat products: black pudding, fatty meat, full-fat sausages, German sausage, haggis, haslet, liver sausage, meat fried in breadcrumbs (e.g. fried beef burgers) meat pies, pasties, pâté (except chicken liver pâté), pork pies, salami, sausages in batter, tongue.

Milk, cream and similar products: butter, cream, double cream, Jersey milk, whipping cream.

Marzipan

Nuts: all nuts except chestnuts, sunflower seeds.

Pasta: pasta served with butter.

Pizza: regular takeaway pizzas.

Poultry: goose, skin from any poultry.

Puddings: chocolate ice-cream, Cornish ice-cream, crème brûlée, gâteaux, pastries, pies, profiteroles with chocolate sauce, roulades, soufflés.

Rice: fried rice.

Sauces: cheese sauce, Hollandaise sauce, sauces made with butter and/or cream.

Snacks: cheeselets and similar biscuits, regular crisps and similar fried snacks, olives, peanuts.

Take-away meals: deep-fat fried foods, meals made with ghee, naan bread.

Vegetables: ackee, avocado, thin or crinkle-cut chips, vegetables served in butter, fried vegetables, vegetables roasted in fat.

8

Recipes

Breakfasts

FRESH FRUIT SMOOTHY

SERVES 1
PER SERVING 342 KCAL/1.9G FAT

1 large ripe banana
175g (6oz) fresh strawberries
150ml (¼ pint) low-fat natural yogurt
150ml (¼ pint) ice cold skimmed milk
1–2 teaspoons runny honey to taste

Peel and slice the banana into a food processor or liquidiser. Remove the tops from the strawberries, slice the strawberries and place in the food processor or liquidiser. Pour in the milk and yogurt and process for a few seconds or until fully combined. Add honey to taste. Pour into a tall glass and serve.

LOW-FAT WAFFLES

MAKES 4

PER WAFFLE 284 KCAL/3G FAT

If you don't have a waffle iron you can use a frying pan instead and place a 12cm (4.5in) cutter inside.

225g (8oz) plain flour
2 tablespoons caster sugar
1 teaspoon baking powder
$1/2$ teaspoon bicarbonate of soda
1 egg
1 teaspoon vanilla extract
300ml ($1/2$ pint) skimmed milk
a little vegetable oil

Combine the flour, sugar, baking powder and bicarbonate of soda in a mixing bowl. Add the egg and vanilla. Using a whisk, gradually pour in the milk, beating the mixture to a smooth, lump-free batter,

Preheat a waffle iron or non-stick frying pan, lightly oil the waffle plate or pan, then remove the oil with kitchen paper.

If using a frying pan, place the cutter in the pan. Spoon 3-4 tablespoons of the mixture into the iron or cutter and cook for 2 minutes. Flip it over and cook the other side for a further 2 minutes. Remove from the pan and keep warm. Repeat with the remaining mixture until you have 4 waffles. Serve hot with jam or marmalade.

QUICK MICROWAVE PORRIDGE WITH DRIED CHERRIES

SERVES 2
PER SERVING 330 KCAL/4.7G FAT

115g (4oz) whole rolled porridge oats
600ml (1 pint) skimmed milk
pinch of salt
25g (1oz) dried cherries or other dried fruit
sugar to taste

Place all the ingredients except the sugar in a large non-metallic bowl and stir well. Cover with clingfilm and microwave on full power for 3 minutes. Remove the clingfilm carefully and stir well. Cover again and cook for a further 3–4 minutes or until thick and creamy. Add sugar to taste and serve.

MUSHROOM FRITTATA

SERVES 2
PER SERVING 167 KCAL/10.5G FAT

225g (8oz) chestnut mushrooms, sliced
4 spring onions, finely chopped
3 eggs
2 tablespoons skimmed milk
1 tablespoon light soy sauce
freshly ground black pepper

Preheat a non-stick frying pan. Add the mushrooms and spring onions and dry-fry for 2–3 minutes until lightly coloured, seasoning well with black pepper.

In a mixing bowl, whisk the eggs, gradually adding the milk and soy sauce. Pour the mixture into a frying pan, reduce the heat and cook gently until the frittata is just set. Fold the frittata in half and slide onto a warmed plate.

SCRAMBLED EGGS WITH SUN-DRIED TOMATOES AND SMOKED SALMON

SERVES 4

PER SERVING 140 KCAL/7.9G FAT

As sun-dried tomatoes are concentrated, they some-times have a salty taste. So, just before serving, taste the dish to check the seasoning and add salt to taste.

6 pieces sun-dried tomatoes (non-oil variety)
4 eggs
2 tablespoons skimmed milk
115g (4oz) smoked salmon, sliced into thin strips
salt and freshly ground black pepper

Microwave method
Slice the sun-dried tomatoes into thin strips and place in a microwave-proof bowl with enough water to barely cover. Cook in the microwave on full power for 4 minutes, drain and return to the bowl.

Break the eggs into the bowl and beat with a fork. Gradually add the milk, beating the mixture until it is fully combined. Season with black pepper and cook in the microwave on high power for 40-second intervals, stirring between cooking, until the egg is just set.

Stir in the smoked salmon strips, and add salt to taste. Serve immediately.

Saucepan method
Slice the sun-dried tomatoes into thin strips and place in a non-stick saucepan. Barely cover with water. Place a lid on the pan and simmer, covered, for 4–5 minutes or until soft.

Combine the eggs, milk and tomatoes in a bowl and pour into the saucepan. Season with black pepper and cook over a low heat, stirring continuously, until the mixture starts to set. Remove from the heat, stir in the smoked salmon and add salt to taste.

POTATO HASH BROWNS

SERVES 4
PER SERVING 132 KCAL/1.9G FAT

450g (1lb) firm waxy potatoes
1 medium onion, finely chopped or grated
2 rashers smoked bacon, finely chopped and
all visible fat removed
salt and freshly ground black pepper

Peel and coarsely grate the potatoes into a mixing bowl. Place them in the centre of a clean dry tea towel, draw together the corners and squeeze tight to remove as much liquid as possible.

Return the potatoes to the bowl and add the onion and bacon. Season well with salt and freshly ground black pepper.

Preheat a non-stick frying pan and add the potato mixture, pressing it down well with a wooden spatula to a depth of approximately 2cm (1in) thick.

Cook, covered, over a low heat for 15 minutes, raise the heat and cook until the mixture forms a crisp base. Flip the potato over and brown on the other side. Slide onto a serving plate and serve immediately

TOASTED CHEESE BAGELS

SERVES 4
PER SERVING 289 KCAL/3.3G FAT

4 virtually fat free bagels
2 tablespoons low-fat quark
2 tablespoons low-fat Cheddar cheese
2 spring onions, finely chopped
1 tablespoon Worcestershire sauce
2 large ripe tomatoes, sliced
salt and black pepper

Preheat a hot grill, slice the bagels in half horizontally and toast lightly on both sides.

In a small bowl, combine the quark, Cheddar cheese, spring onions and Worcestershire sauce. Season well with salt and black pepper.

Spread the mixture onto the bagel halves and arrange slices of tomato on top. Return to the grill until golden brown.

Lunches

CORONATION CHICKEN

SERVES 4
PER SERVING 287 KCAL/3.2G FAT

4 skinned and boned chicken breasts, cooked
225g (8oz) virtually fat free fromage frais
1 tablespoon curry powder
2 tablespoons mango chutney
225g (8oz) seedless grapes
2 tablespoons lemon juice
1 tablespoon chopped fresh parsley
salt and freshly ground black pepper
bunch of watercress to serve

Coarsely chop the cooked chicken and place in a mixing bowl.

Blend together the fromage frais, curry powder and mango chutney. Mix with the chicken, coating it well.

Cut the grapes in half with a sharp knife, add to the chicken and combine all the ingredients well. At this point you can leave the dish to stand or store it in the refrigerator until ready to serve.

Just before serving, mix in the lemon juice and the parsley and season well with salt and pepper.

Serve with a watercress salad.

PRAWN AND PASTA SALAD

SERVES 4
PER SERVING 255 KCAL/2.2G FAT

450g (1lb) [cooked weight] pasta shells
450g (1lb) peeled and cooked prawns
150g (5oz) low-fat natural yogurt
1 tablespoon tomato purée
a few drops Tabasco sauce to taste
3 spring onions, chopped

Combine the cooked pasta shells and prawns in a serving bowl.

In a small bowl stir together the yogurt, tomato purée and Tabasco sauce. Pour onto the pasta mixture and toss well.

Just before serving, sprinkle with the spring onions. Serve either at room temperature or slightly chilled.

THAI NOODLE SALAD

SERVES 2
PER SERVING 212 KCAL/0.4G FAT

115g (4oz) [dry weight] vermicelli rice noodles
1 small red onion, finely diced
4 ripe tomatoes, skinned, seeded and finely diced
1/2 cucumber, peeled and cut into julienne strips
zest and juice of 1 lime
1 red chilli, seeded and finely chopped
2 tablespoons chopped fresh coriander

for the dressing
2 tablespoons fresh apple juice
2 tablespoons fresh lime juice
1 teaspoon sugar
2 teaspoons Thai fish sauce or oyster sauce
salt and freshly ground black pepper

Cook the noodles according to the packet instructions. Drain and rinse well.

Place the onion, tomatoes and cucumber in a large mixing bowl. Add the noodles, lime zest and juice, chilli and coriander and mix well. Divide the mixture equally between 2 serving bowls.

Combine the dressing ingredients in a bowl and pour over the salad.

POTATO AND WATERCRESS SALAD

SERVES 6
PER SERVING 129 KCAL/2.4G FAT

450–675g (1–1½lb) new potatoes
115g (4oz) lean back bacon
4 spring onions or 2 tablespoons chopped fresh chives
1 bunch fresh watercress
1 tablespoon chopped fresh parsley

for the dressing
150g (5oz) low-fat natural yogurt
2–3 teaspoons French mustard
1 teaspoon caster sugar or artificial sweetener to taste
1 tablespoon white wine vinegar
salt and freshly ground black pepper

Scrub baby potatoes and cook whole, or scrape large ones and cut into pieces. Cook in boiling salted water until just tender. Drain well and place under cold running water until completely cold. Drain well. If using large potatoes cut them into dice.

In the meantime, remove any fat from the bacon and grill the rashers until they are crisp. Drain on kitchen paper.

Trim and slice the spring onions. Coarsely chop the watercress. Place the potatoes in a bowl with the spring onions or chives and the watercress. Crush the bacon into small pieces and sprinkle into the mixture.

Mix together all the ingredients for the dressing and taste to check the seasoning. Pour over the potatoes and mix well. Sprinkle with the chopped parsley, cover and refrigerate until required.

CURRIED CHICKEN AND YOGURT SALAD

SERVES 1
PER SERVING 186 KCAL/2.9G FAT

150g (5oz) low-fat natural yogurt
1 teaspoon curry powder
75g (3oz) cooked chicken breast, cut into cubes
unlimited green salad vegetables

Mix the yogurt and curry powder together in a bowl. Add the chicken and stir well. Serve on a bed of fresh green salad vegetables.

QUICK TUNA PATE

SERVES 1
PER SERVING 276 KCAL/2.8G FAT

200g (7oz) tinned tuna in brine
75g (3oz) low-fat yogurt
2 tablespoons reduced-oil salad dressing
2 teaspoons lemon juice
1 teaspoon chopped fresh or freeze-dried dill
¼ teaspoon cayenne pepper
1 lemon slice
salt and freshly ground black pepper

Drain the tuna well and place in a bowl. Add the yogurt, reduced-oil dressing and lemon juice. Mash with a fork until well combined. Add the fresh dill and cayenne pepper and season well with salt and pepper. Mix well.

Spoon the mixture into a dish and place a slice of lemon on top. Refrigerate for at least 2 hours before serving.

POTTED SMOKED TROUT

SERVES 2
PER SERVING 192 KCAL/6.4G FAT

225g (8oz) fresh smoked trout fillets
1 tablespoon Dijon mustard
115g (4oz) quark
1 tablespoon chopped fresh parsley
salt and freshly ground black pepper
1 bunch watercress

Using a fork, break the trout fillets in a small bowl. Add the mustard, quark, and parsley. Mix well, and season with salt and pepper.

Press the mixture into 2 dishes and smooth the tops over with a knife.

Refrigerate until ready to serve. Just before serving, garnish with watercress.

FRENCH ONION SOUP

SERVES 4
PER SERVING 190 KCAL/2.4G FAT

675g (1½lb) large onions, sliced
1.2 litres (2 pints) vegetable stock
2 garlic cloves, crushed
1 tablespoon chopped fresh thyme
2 tablespoons plain flour
salt and freshly ground black pepper
2 tablespoons chopped fresh parsley
2 slices bread, toasted and cut into croutons

Place the onions in a large pan with a little vegetable stock. Sweat the onions until soft. Add the garlic and thyme. Sprinkle the flour over and mix well. Season to taste, and cook for 1 minute to cook out the flour. Gradually add the remaining stock, bring to the boil and simmer for 10 minutes.

Just before serving, sprinkle with the parsley and toasted croutons.

DOUBLE SOUP OF RED AND YELLOW PEPPERS

SERVES 4
PER SERVING 194 KCAL/2.3G FAT

6 red peppers, seeded and chopped
6 yellow peppers, seeded and chopped
2 large onions, chopped
2 garlic cloves, crushed
2 teaspoons chopped fresh thyme
2 celery sticks, chopped
2.5 litres (4 pints) vegetable stock
2 bay leaves
salt and freshly ground black pepper
sprig of parsley or a little fromage frais to garnish

Using 2 separate pans, place the red peppers in one and the yellow peppers in the other. Divide all the other ingredients, except the parsley or fromage frais, in half and place half in each pan. Cover with a lid and simmer for 20–25 minutes or until soft.

Remove the bay leaf from each pan and pour one mixture into a liquidiser or food processor. Blend until smooth, then pour into a clean pan to reheat. Rinse out the liquidiser or food processor and repeat with the second mixture, pouring it into a separate pan when blended.

To serve, pour equal quantities of each soup into 2 separate jugs. Holding a jug in each hand at either side of a soup bowl, pour both soups into the bowl.

Garnish with a sprig of parsley or a swirl of fromage frais.

PUMPKIN AND GINGER SOUP

SERVES 2
PER SERVING 144 KCAL/2G FAT

2 medium onions, diced
2 garlic cloves, crushed
450g (1lb) pumpkin, peeled and seeds removed
2 tablespoons chopped fresh ginger
1 tablespoon chopped fresh thyme
1.5 litres (2½ pints) chicken stock
2 tablespoons tomato purée
salt and freshly ground black pepper
low-fat natural yogurt and chopped fresh parsley to garnish

Dry-fry the onions and garlic in a non-stick saucepan until soft. Add the pumpkin and ginger and cook for a further 2–3 minutes, taking care not to allow the ginger to brown. Add the thyme and stock. Bring to the boil and simmer for 25–30 minutes until tender.

Place the soup in a liquidiser or food processor and blend until smooth. Return to the saucepan and stir in the tomato purée. Season with salt and freshly ground black pepper. Adjust the consistency with a little stock or skimmed milk.

Just before serving, garnish with a swirl of yogurt and a little chopped parsley.

CHUNKY VEGETABLE SOUP

SERVES 3
'PER SERVING 154 KCAL/2.2G FAT

2 small carrots, thinly sliced
2 leeks, thinly sliced
1–2 parsnips, cut into 5mm ($\frac{1}{4}$in) dice
1–2 celery sticks, thinly sliced
1 medium onion, thinly sliced
$\frac{1}{4}$–$\frac{1}{2}$ medium swede, cut into 5mm ($\frac{1}{4}$in) dice
a few dark green cabbage leaves, chopped
1 × 400g (14oz) tin chopped tomatoes
1 garlic clove, crushed
1 bay leaf
2 level teaspoons salt
1–2 litres (2–3 pints) vegetable stock
50g (2oz) [dry weight] small pasta shapes
1 level teaspoon dried oregano (optional)
black pepper to taste

Place all the vegetables and the chopped tomatoes in a very large pan. Add the garlic, bay leaf, salt and vegetable stock. Bring to the boil and simmer for 20 minutes, until the vegetables are tender.

Add the pasta shapes and dried oregano and cook for a further 20 minutes.

When the soup is cooked, remove the bay leaf and discard. Season to taste. If a thick soup is preferred, place half the vegetables in a liquidiser, purée, then stir back into the remaining vegetables.

CARAMELISED ONION AND LEMON SOUP WITH CHIVE AND PARSLEY CREAM

SERVES 4
PER SERVING 156 KCAL/1.6G FAT

1kg (2¼lb) cooking onions, thinly sliced
1 teaspoon caster sugar
4 garlic cloves, crushed
1 tablespoon chopped fresh thyme
zest and juice of 1 lemon
2 tablespoons plain flour
1.2 litres (2 pints) vegetable stock
150ml (¼ pint) low-fat natural yogurt
1 tablespoon chopped fresh chives
1 tablespoon chopped fresh flat leaf parsley
salt and freshly ground black pepper
1 lemon to garnish

In a large non-stick saucepan, dry-fry the onions with the sugar for 4–5 minutes until they start to caramelise and turn brown. Add the garlic, thyme and lemon zest and juice, sprinkle the flour over and mix in well with a wooden spoon. Cook over a low heat, stirring well for 1 minute in order to cook out the flour.

Gradually add the stock, stirring well to prevent any lumps from forming. Bring to the boil and then reduce the heat and simmer for 20 minutes.

Taste and season with salt and freshly ground black pepper. Just before serving, combine the herbs with the yogurt. Serve the soup hot in warmed bowls and garnish with a slice of lemon and a swirl of chive and parsley cream.

SMOKED FISH AND CORN CHOWDER

SERVES 4
PER SERVING 252 KCAL/2G FAT

450g (1lb) smoked haddock or cod
2 onions, chopped
2 tablespoons plain flour
2 teaspoons English mustard powder
225g (8oz) tinned sweetcorn, drained
225g (8oz) potatoes, peeled and cut into 1cm ($\frac{1}{2}$in) dice
600ml (1 pint) fish stock
300ml ($\frac{1}{2}$ pint) skimmed milk
2 tablespoons chopped fresh parsley
2 tablespoons virtually fat free fromage frais
salt and freshly ground black pepper

Place the fish in a saucepan. Add 600ml (1 pint) of water and simmer for 10 minutes until tender. Drain, reserving the liquid. Flake the fish coarsely, discarding any skin and bones.

Dry-fry the onions in a large non-stick pan until soft. Add 3 tablespoons of the reserved liquid, sprinkle the flour over and beat well with a wooden spoon. Cook for 1 minute in order to cook out the flour. Gradually add the rest of the reserved liquid, stirring continuously. Add the mustard powder, sweetcorn and potatoes, stock and milk. Bring to the boil, reduce the heat and simmer for 10 minutes until the vegetables are tender. Stir in the flaked fish and the parsley. Taste, and adjust the seasoning with a fish stock cube if necessary and salt and pepper. Just before serving, stir in the fromage frais.

BEEF STROGANOFF

SERVES 6
PER SERVING 217 KCAL/7.2G FAT

1 medium onion, finely chopped
2 garlic cloves, crushed
675g (1½lb) lean beef fillet, sliced
1 tablespoon plain flour
1 wineglass white wine
150ml (¼ pint) beef stock
1 tablespoon Dijon mustard
225g (8oz) button mushrooms, sliced
300ml (½ pint) low-fat natural yogurt
2 tablespoons chopped fresh parsley
salt and freshly ground black pepper
pinch of paprika

Preheat a non-stick wok or frying pan. Dry-fry the onion until soft. Add the garlic and the beef, season well and cook until sealed.

Sprinkle the flour over the beef. Stir well and cook for 1 minute to cook out the flour.

Add the white wine and the stock and mix well. Stir in the mustard and mushrooms and simmer for 2–3 minutes until the sauce thickens.

Remove the pan from the heat and stir in the yogurt and parsley. Check the seasoning. Just before serving, dust with paprika.

VEGETABLE CROQUETTES

SERVES 1
PER SERVING 405 KCAL/9.5G FAT

115g (4oz) mashed potatoes
50g (2oz) sage and onion stuffing mix
115g (4oz) any frozen mixed vegetables
1 small onion, grated
salt and freshly ground black pepper
1 egg, beaten
breadcrumbs to coat

Preheat the oven to 180C, 350F, Gas Mark 4. Bind all the ingredients together, using half of the beaten egg.

Shape the mixture into croquettes. Dip the croquettes in the remaining egg and roll in the breadcrumbs. Place on a non-stick baking tray and bake in the oven for 15 minutes or until golden brown.

PASTA WITH SPINACH SAUCE

SERVES 1
PER SERVING 334 KCAL/3.3G FAT

50g (2oz) [dry weight] wholemeal fusilli pasta
300g (12oz) fresh spinach or 150g (6oz) frozen spinach
115g (4oz) quark
salt and freshly ground black pepper
a little fromage frais or skimmed milk

Cook the pasta as directed and drain well.

Wash the fresh spinach (if using) and cook in 1 table-spoon of water. Drain well and chop finely in a food processor or with a knife. If using frozen spinach, cook as directed.

Mix the quark with the spinach, and add salt and pepper to taste. If the mixture is too stiff, add a little low-fat fromage frais or skimmed milk.

Heat the spinach sauce, add the cooked pasta and pile onto a serving plate.

SMOKED HAM MACARONI CHEESE

SERVES 4
324 KCAL/4.8G FAT

225g (8oz) [dry weight] macaroni pasta
300ml (½ pint) skimmed milk
1 tablespoon vegetable stock powder or
1 vegetable stock cube
4 teaspoons cornflour
1 tablespoon Dijon mustard
50g (2oz) low fat Cheddar cheese, grated
115g (4oz) thinly sliced smoked ham, cut into strips
1 tablespoon chopped fresh chives
salt and freshly ground black pepper

Preheat the oven to 190C, 375F, Gas Mark 5. Cook the pasta in boiling salted water until tender. Drain through a colander and rinse under cold water to prevent further cooking.

In a saucepan, heat the milk and the stock. Mix the cornflour with a little cold water and stir into the sauce.

Stir continuously as the sauce thickens, then reduce the heat and simmer for 2–3 minutes.

Stir in the remaining ingredients and season well with salt and pepper. Add the cooked pasta and mix well. Pour into an ovenproof dish. Bake in the oven for 20 minutes until golden brown.

THE ULTIMATE BLT

SERVES 1
PER SERVING 312 KCAL/8.5G FAT

2 rashers bacon, all visible fat removed
2–3 leaves romaine or crisp lettuce
2–3 sweet cherry tomatoes
2–3 cornichons or 1 pickled baby gherkin
1 tablespoon low-fat salad dressing
1 tablespoon tomato ketchup
$\frac{1}{4}$ teaspoon cayenne pepper
2 slices medium-cut white or brown bread

Preheat the grill on the highest setting. Place the bacon on a wire rack over a grill tray and cook under a hot grill on each side. Remove and place on a kitchen paper to absorb any remaining fat.

Shred the lettuce, slice the tomatoes and cornichons or baby gherkin. In a small bowl, mix together the salad dressing, ketchup and cayenne pepper and spread onto both slices of bread. Place the lettuce on the bottom of one slice, followed by the bacon and then the tomatoes and cornichons or gherkin. Place the remaining slice of bread on top and press down lightly. Cut in half and serve.

SEAFOOD PANCAKES WITH MUSTARD SAUCE

SERVES 4

PER SERVING 330 KCAL/6G FAT

115g (4oz) plain flour
pinch of salt
1 egg
300ml (½ pint) skimmed milk
1 tablespoon finely chopped fresh parsley
4 teaspoons vegetable oil (to line the pan)

for the filling
450g (1lb) mixed cooked seafood (mussels,
prawns, crab, smoked fish)
1 onion, finely chopped
150ml (¼ pint) fish stock
2 tablespoons plain flour
300ml (½ pint) skimmed milk
1 teaspoon Dijon mustard
1 teaspoon freshly chopped dill
salt and black pepper

Make the pancake batter by sifting the flour and salt into a large bowl or jug. Add the egg and a little milk and stir into the flour to make a thick paste, beating well to remove any lumps. Gradually add the remaining milk and the parsley. Beat to a smooth consistency, then allow to stand for 20 minutes.

Prepare the fish and seafood, removing any skin and bones, and combine in a bowl.

In a non-stick saucepan, dry-fry the onion until soft. Add 2 tablespoons of the fish stock and the flour and cook for 1 minute, stirring with a wooden spoon, to allow the flour to cook out. Gradually add the remaining stock and milk, stirring continuously to prevent any lumps forming. Bring to the boil and allow to thicken. Stir the mustard and dill into the sauce and season well with salt and black pepper. Add half of the sauce to the seafood and mix well.

Preheat the oven to 190C, 375F, Gas Mark 5. Preheat a non-stick frying pan. Add 1 teaspoon of oil, then wipe out with kitchen paper, taking care not to burn your fingers (wear an oven glove if necessary).

Whisk the batter well, then add 2 tablespoons to the pan, tilting the pan to allow the batter to coat the base. Cook briskly for 30 seconds then loosen the edges with a wooden spatula, flip the pancake over and cook the other side for 15 seconds and slide onto a plate. Repeat until you have 8 pancakes, adding oil to the pan and wiping out after every 2 pancakes.

Place a pancake in a large ovenproof dish, add 2 spoonfuls of seafood mixture then fold over and place at one end of the dish. Repeat with the remaining pancakes, then spoon the remaining sauce on top.

Place in the oven for 30 minutes.

ITALIAN TOAST TOPPERS

SERVES 2

PER SERVING 248 KCAL/2.6G FAT

4 slices medium-cut white or brown bread
1 medium onion, thinly sliced
1 red pepper, seeded and finely sliced

2 garlic cloves, crushed
1 courgette, finely sliced
115g (4oz) chestnut mushrooms, sliced
1 × 200g (7oz) tin chopped tomatoes
1 tablespoon chopped fresh oregano
salt and freshly ground black pepper

Toast the bread on both sides very lightly and set aside.

Preheat a non-stick frying pan, and dry-fry the onion for 2–3 minutes until soft. Add the red pepper, garlic, courgette and mushrooms and cook briskly over a high heat, turning them over regularly.

Stir in the tomatoes and oregano and simmer gently for 5–6 minutes until the liquid has reduced to leave a thick, chunky paste. Spread the mixture onto the toasted bread and place under a hot grill for 2–3 minutes to brown. Serve hot.

BAKED GINGER STUFFED TOMATOES

SERVES 2
PER SERVING 129 KCAL/1.6G FAT

4 large ripe beef tomatoes
1 medium onion, finely diced
1 red pepper, seeded and diced
2 garlic cloves, crushed
1 tablespoon fresh ginger, skinned and finely chopped
1 × 200g (7oz) tin chopped tomatoes
1 tablespoon chopped chervil
salt and freshly ground black pepper

Preheat the oven to 190C, 375F, Gas Mark 5. Slice off the tops of the tomatoes and reserve. Using a dessertspoon, remove the inner core and seeds from the tomatoes. Place the tomato shells in an ovenproof dish.

Preheat a non-stick frying pan and dry-fry the onion for 2–3 minutes until soft. Add the pepper, garlic and ginger and cook for a further 2–3 minutes. Stir in the chopped tomatoes and chervil and simmer until the sauce thickens, seasoning well with salt and black pepper. Spoon the cooked mixture into the tomato shells and place a tomato top over each one. Bake in the oven for 20 minutes. Serve hot or cold.

SPINACH SOUFFLE

SERVES 2
PER SERVING 238 KCAL/8.6G FAT

300ml (½ pint) skimmed milk
1 tablespoon vegetable stock powder or 1 vegetable
stock cube
4 teaspoons cornflour
1 tablespoon Dijon mustard
225g (8oz) baby leaf spinach
2 egg yolks
4 egg whites
salt and freshly ground black pepper
grated fresh nutmeg

Preheat the oven to 190C, 350F, Gas Mark 5. Prepare 4 individual 115g (4oz) ramekin dishes by lightly greasing the insides with a little vegetable oil and then removing the excess with a piece of kitchen paper.

Heat the milk and stock in a saucepan. Slake the cornflour with a little water and stir into the milk, stirring continuously as the sauce thickens. Reduce the heat and simmer for 2–3 minutes. Mix in the mustard and spinach and allow the mixture to cool.

When the mixture is quite cool, beat in the egg yolks and season with salt and black pepper.

Whisk the egg whites until they form stiff peaks. Using a large metal spoon, gently fold a third of the egg whites into the cooled mixture until combined, then fold in the remaining egg white. Spoon the mixture into the prepared ramekin dishes and sprinkle the grated nutmeg on top.

Bake in the oven for 20–25 minutes until well risen and golden brown. Serve immediately.

CRUNCHY BACON AND SPAGHETTI

SERVES 1
PER SERVING 357 KCAL/2.5G FAT

3 thin slices lean smoked bacon
50g (2oz) [dry weight] wholemeal spaghetti
1 small tin chopped tomatoes
2 medium mushrooms, thinly sliced
2 tablespoons frozen sweetcorn
1 tablespoon Branston pickle
2 teaspoons cornflour
salt and pepper to taste

Trim any visible fat from the bacon. Grill the bacon on both sides.

Cook the spaghetti in boiling salted water for 10 minutes. While the spaghetti is cooking, place the tomatoes in a saucepan and add the mushrooms, sweetcorn and pickle. Cook on a moderate heat, then allow to simmer.

Wipe off any traces of fat from the bacon with kitchen paper, then snip into bite-size pieces and add to the tomato mixture.

Dissolve the cornflour in a little cold water and gradually add to the bacon and tomato mixture so that it thicken it as it simmers. Season to taste.

By the time the spaghetti is cooked, the bacon and tomato mixture will be ready to serve. Drain the spaghetti, place on a serving plate and top with the bacon and tomato mixture.

TUNA AND TARRAGON PASTA

SERVES 1
PER SERVING 389 KCAL/2.6G FAT

50g (2oz) [dry weight] wholewheat pasta
1 × 185g (6½oz) tin tuna in brine
1 tablespoon chopped fresh tarragon
1 tablespoon tarragon vinegar or cider vinegar
1 tablespoon tomato ketchup
1 tomato, chopped
50g (2oz) tinned peas, drained
50g (2oz) tinned sweetcorn, drained
freshly ground black pepper

Cook the pasta in boiling salted water for 8 minutes.

Meanwhile, drain and flake the tuna and mix with the chopped tarragon, the tarragon or cider vinegar and the tomato ketchup.

Place the tomato, peas, sweetcorn and tuna and tarragon mixture in a saucepan. Mix well and heat thoroughly.

Drain the pasta and top with the tuna sauce. Serve with a generous grinding of freshly ground black pepper.

CHEESY STUFFED POTATO

SERVES 1
PER SERVING 208 KCAL/5.3G FAT

1 medium potato, baked in its jacket
50g (2oz) low-fat cottage cheese
25g (1oz) low-fat Cheddar cheese
1 teaspoon Dijon mustard
3 tablespoons skimmed milk
salt and freshly ground black pepper
pinch of paprika

Preheat the oven to 180C, 375F, Gas Mark 5. Cut the pre-cooked potato in half lengthways and carefully scoop out the pulp with a spoon, leaving a 5mm (¼in) shell.

Place the potato pulp in a large bowl. Add the cheeses, mustard and skimmed milk and season to taste. Mash with a fork or potato masher until the mixture is well blended. Spoon the mixture into the empty potato shell, sprinkle with paprika and bake in the oven for 15–20 minutes.

FRENCH BREAD PIZZA

SERVES 1
PER SERVING 252 KCAL/2.8G FAT

1 × 50g (2oz) French stick
200g (7oz) tinned chopped tomatoes or
3 tablespoons tomato purée
1 onion, finely chopped
25g (1oz) ham, chopped
$\frac{1}{2}$ red or green pepper, chopped
50g (2oz) pineapple, chopped
4 mushrooms, chopped
sprinkling of mixed herbs

Cut the French stick in half lengthways.

If using tinned tomatoes, boil them in a pan to reduce them. Spread the tinned tomatoes or tomato purée on the bread and top with the chopped onion, ham, red or green pepper, pineapple and mushrooms. Sprinkle the mixed herbs on top.

Place under the grill and grill under a moderate heat for 5–6 minutes, until the topping goes slightly brown and the bread is crispy.

CLUB SANDWICH

SERVES 1
PER SERVING 413 KCAL/10G FAT

50g (2oz) lean bacon
3 slices bread
1 teaspoon reduced-oil salad dressing
1 teaspoon tomato ketchup
$\frac{1}{2}$ teaspoon mustard
25g (1oz) cooked chicken
1 tomato
shredded lettuce leaves
4 cocktail sticks

Grill the bacon until well cooked and crisp.

Toast the bread. Spread one slice with reduced-oil dressing, the second slice with tomato ketchup and the third with mustard.

Cut the chicken and tomato into slices and place on the first slice of toast. Place the toast spread with ketchup on top of this, then add the bacon followed by shredded lettuce. Top with the remaining piece of toast (spread with mustard). Press together firmly. Cut into 4 triangles crossways and pierce each piece with a cocktail stick to hold it together.

Dinners

Meat and poultry

ROAST BEEF WITH YORKSHIRE PUDDING, DRY-ROAST POTATOES AND PARSNIPS

SERVES 6

PER SERVING BEEF: 218 KCAL/8.3G FAT; DRY-ROAST
POTATOES AND PARSNIPS: 106 KCAL/0.9G FAT;
YORKSHIRE PUDDING: 79 KCAL/1.3G FAT

1 × 900g (2lb) joint lean beef (topside)
1 onion, finely diced
1 carrot, diced
1 celery stick, diced
2 teaspoons mixed dried herbs
600ml (1 pint) beef stock
1 tablespoon cornflour
1–2 drops gravy browning

for the dry-roast potatoes and parsnips
450g (1lb) potatoes, peeled and cut in half
8 medium parsnips, peeled and left whole
1 tablespoon soy sauce diluted in 2 tablespoons water
(optional)

for the Yorkshire pudding batter
115g (4oz) plain flour
1 egg
pinch of salt
150ml (¼ pint) skimmed milk

Preheat the oven to 180C, 350F, Gas Mark 4. Prepare the beef by removing as much visible fat as possible.

Place the onion, carrot, celery and herbs in the bottom of a roasting tin or ovenproof dish, sit the beef on top and pour 300ml (½ pint) water around. Place in the oven. Allow 15 minutes per 450g (1lb) plus 15 minutes over for rare beef, 20 minutes per 450g (1lb) plus 20 minutes over for medium rare, and 25 minutes per 450g (1lb) plus 30 minutes over if you like your beef well done.

Cook the potatoes and parsnips separately in boiling water. Drain and place in a non-stick roasting tin. Place in the top of the oven for 35–40 minutes until golden brown. You can baste the vegetables with the diluted soy sauce if they appear to dry out.

Forty minutes before the beef is ready, make the batter by blending the flour with the egg and a little milk to a smooth paste. Add the salt and whisk in the remaining milk until smooth. Preheat a 6-hole, non-stick Yorkshire pudding tin for 2 minutes in the oven. Remove and half-fill each mould with batter. Increase the oven temperature to 200C, 400F, Gas Mark 6, place the pudding batter in the oven and cook for 35–40 minutes.

When the beef is cooked, remove it from the roasting tin and wrap in foil to keep warm. Allow it to rest for 5–10 minutes. Meanwhile, add the beef stock to the pan juices, slake the cornflour with a little water and add to the pan. Stir well as the gravy thickens and add 1–2 drops of gravy browning as required.

To serve, carve the beef thinly. Serve with the Yorkshire puddings, dry-roast potatoes and parsnips, gravy and seasonal vegetables.

BEEF AND PEPPER SKEWERS WITH TERIYAKI SAUCE

SERVES 2
PER SERVING 294 KCAL/9.2G FAT

350g (12oz) extra thin beef steaks
1 green pepper, seeded and cut into chunks

for the sauce
4 tablespoons soy sauce
4 tablespoons dry sherry
1 garlic clove, crushed
1 teaspoon ground ginger
1 teaspoon dark Muscovado sugar

Cut the steaks into thin strips, then thread the strips, concertina-style, onto 4 large skewers, placing a chunk of green pepper between each strip.

To make the sauce, place all the ingredients in a small pan and heat gently until simmering, stirring occasionally. Allow the sauce to simmer gently while you cook the meat.

Place the skewers on a grill pan and brush a little sauce over the meat and peppers. Cook under a pre-heated grill for 5–8 minutes, basting occasionally with a little more of the sauce.

When cooked, arrange the skewers on a plate and pour the remaining sauce over the meat.

STEAK AND KIDNEY PIE

SERVES 4

PER SERVING 355 KCAL/6.8G FAT

225g (8oz) lean rump or sirloin steak
225g (8oz) kidneys, cut into bite-sized pieces
2 medium onions, chopped
1 wineglass red wine
2 beef stock cubes
1 tablespoon gravy powder
900g (2lb) potatoes, peeled
2 tablespoons low-fat natural yogurt
4–5 tablespoons skimmed milk
salt and freshly ground black pepper

Preheat the oven to 180C, 350F, Gas Mark 4. Trim the steak, removing all visible fat, then cut the steak into cubes. Preheat a non-stick frying pan. Dry-fry the cubes of beef steak and kidneys until well browned. Place in a 12×8in (30×20cm) pie dish. Dry-fry the onion until soft and add this to the meat in the pie dish.

Place 300ml (½ pint) water in the pan. Add the wine and stock cubes and bring to the boil. Mix the gravy powder with a little cold water and add to the boiling stock in the pan, stirring continuously. The gravy should be quite thick. Add more gravy powder mixed with a little water as necessary. Pour the gravy over the meat in the pie dish.

Boil the potatoes and drain. Mash the potatoes with the yogurt and sufficient skimmed milk to make the consistency quite soft. Season to taste. Using a fork or a piping bag with a star nozzle, carefully spoon or pipe the potato on top of the meat and gravy, spreading the potato so that it covers the meat completely.

Place in the oven and cook for 30–40 minutes, or until crisp and brown on top.

PEPPERED STEAK WITH CHIVE AND TARRAGON SAUCE

SERVES 4

PER SERVING 374 KCAL/14.1G FAT

4 × 225g (4 × 8oz) lean fillet steaks
8 tablespoons mixed peppercorns (green,
black, red and white)
1 good tablespoon plain flour
300ml (½ pint) skimmed milk
1 tablespoon vegetable stock powder or 1 vegetable
stock cube
1 teaspoon Dijon mustard
1 tablespoon finely chopped fresh chives
1 tablespoon finely chopped fresh tarragon
sea salt

Preheat the grill on the highest setting. Prepare the steaks by removing any visible fat. Using the palms of your hands, gently flatten the steaks (this will help them to cook more quickly). Place to one side.

Crush the peppercorns either in a pestle and mortar or by placing them on a chopping board and crushing them with the broad edge of a heavy chopping knife. Place onto a flat plate.

Season both sides of each steak generously with salt, then dip both sides of each steak into the peppercorns, pressing the peppercorns well into the meat. Place the steaks on a non-stick baking tray and cook under a hot grill to your liking (2–3 minutes each side for rare, 3–4 minutes each side for medium, and 5–6 minutes each side for well done).

When the steaks are almost ready, strain off the meat juices collected on the baking tray into a saucepan. Add the flour and cook over a low heat for 1 minute in order to cook out the flour. Gradually add the milk and stock, stirring continuously to prevent lumps from forming. Add the mustard and herbs and simmer gently.

Place the steaks onto a serving dish and pour the sauce on top.

COTTAGE PIE WITH LEEK AND POTATO TOPPING

SERVES 4
PER SERVING 359 KCAL/8G FAT

450g (1lb) lean minced beef
1 onion, chopped
2 carrots, chopped
2 tablespoons plain flour
300ml (½ pint) beef stock
1 tablespoon tomato purée
1 tablespoon mixed dried herbs
salt and freshly ground black pepper

for the topping
675g (1½lb) potatoes, peeled and chopped
2 leeks, sliced
2 tablespoons skimmed milk
50g (2oz) low-fat Cheddar cheese, grated
salt and freshly ground black pepper

Preheat the oven to 190C, 375F, Gas Mark 5. Boil the potatoes until softened, adding the leeks 5 minutes before the end of cooking.

Meanwhile, dry-fry the mince for 3–4 minutes in a non-stick frying pan. Remove the mince from the pan and drain. Discard the liquid and put the meat to one side. Wipe out the pan. Return the meat to the pan. Add the onion and carrots and stir in the flour. Gradually add the stock, tomato purée and dried herbs. Bring to the boil and stir until thickened. Season with salt and black pepper. Transfer to an ovenproof dish.

Drain the potatoes and leeks and mash with a little milk and half the cheese. Season to taste. Place on top of the mince mixture. Sprinkle with the remaining cheese.

Bake in the oven for 25 minutes until golden.

BEEF AND MUSHROOM CANNELLONI

SERVES 4
PER SERVING 353 KCAL/12.5G FAT

1 large onion, finely diced
450g (1lb) lean minced beef
2 garlic cloves, crushed

225g (8oz) chestnut mushrooms, finely sliced
1 tablespoon mushroom soy or dark soy sauce
2 beef stock cubes
1 × 400g (14oz) tin chopped tomatoes
2 tablespoons tomato purée
2 tablespoons chopped fresh oregano or marjoram
8 lasagne sheets
salt and freshly ground black pepper

for the topping
300ml (½ pint) virtually fat free Normandy fromage frais
115g (4oz) chestnut mushrooms, very finely chopped
1 teaspoon English mustard powder
1 tablespoon white wine
salt and black pepper

Preheat the oven to 200C, 400F, Gas Mark 6. Dry-fry the onion in a non-stick pan until soft, add the beef and garlic and cook over a high heat for 5–6 minutes.

Add the mushrooms and soy sauce, then crumble the stock cubes over the top. Add the chopped tomatoes, purée and herbs, and simmer for 15–20 minutes.

Meanwhile, cook the lasagne sheets in plenty of salted water until just cooked. Drain and cover with cold water to prevent further cooking. Drain the lasagne again and lay the sheets out flat. Season well with salt and pepper. Place one sheet in an ovenproof dish and cover the centre (about a third of the sheet) with some of the beef mixture. Roll up the sheet into a cylindrical shape and place at one end of the dish. Repeat with the remaining sheets and mixture and pour any leftover mixture over the top.

Combine all the topping ingredients and season to taste. Pour over the top of the cannelloni. Bake in the oven for 25–30 minutes.

SPAGHETTI BOLOGNESE

SERVES 4

PER SERVING 495 KCAL/12.7G FAT

450g (1lb) lean minced beef
2 garlic cloves, crushed
1 large onion, finely chopped
2 medium carrots, finely grated
2 beef stock cubes
2 x 400g (2 x 14oz) tins chopped tomatoes
4 tablespoons tomato purée
1 tablespoon chopped fresh oregano or
1 teaspoon dried oregano
1 vegetable stock cube
350g (12oz) [dry weight] spaghetti
salt and freshly ground black pepper
chopped fresh herbs to garnish

Dry-fry the minced beef in a non-stick pan until it starts to change colour. Remove the mince from the pan and drain through a colander. Wipe out the pan with kitchen paper.

Return the meat to the pan, add the garlic and onion and continue cooking for a further 2–3 minutes, stirring well. Add the carrots and crumble the beef stock cubes over the top. Add the tomatoes, tomato purée and oregano and mix well to allow the stock cubes to dissolve. Reduce the heat to a gentle simmer, season well with black pepper, cover with a lid and continue to simmer gently for 30 minutes until the sauce thickens.

Meanwhile, bring a large pan of salted water to the boil and add the vegetable stock cube. Add the spaghetti and cook until the spaghetti is soft but slightly firm in the centre. Drain through a colander.

Arrange the spaghetti on warmed plates, pour the sauce on top and garnish with fresh herbs.

PAN-FRIED LIVER WITH ONIONS AND BALSAMIC VINEGAR

SERVES 2
PER SERVING 354 KCAL/12.8G FAT

1 teaspoon vegetable oil
1 tablespoon plain flour
450g (1lb) lamb's liver
1 medium onion, finely diced
1 teaspoon ground coriander
3 tablespoons balsamic vinegar
150ml (¼ pint) lamb stock
salt and freshly ground black pepper

Place the oil in a non-stick frying pan and heat the pan. Wipe out the pan with kitchen paper, taking care not to burn your fingers (wear an oven glove if necessary).

Season the flour with salt and pepper and toss the liver in it so that it is well coated. Place the liver in the hot pan to seal on both sides (this will take about 1–2 minutes each side depending on how thick the slices are).

Remove the liver from the pan and place in a low oven (150C, 300F, Gas Mark 2) to continue cooking. Place the onion and coriander in the frying pan and dry-fry until the onion softens. Add the balsamic vinegar.

To de-glaze the pan, stir in the stock, scraping any residue from the pan. Just before serving, return the liver to the pan to coat with the sauce.

LAMB BURGERS

SERVES 4
PER SERVING 237 KCAL/6.8G FAT

450g (1lb) lean minced lamb
1 small onion, finely chopped
2 tablespoons tomato ketchup
salt and freshly ground black pepper

Mix all the ingredients together and season well with salt and pepper.

Divide the mixture into 4 portions and form into burger shapes.

Cook each burger under a very hot grill or on a barbecue for 5–6 minutes on each side.

GRILLED MARINATED LAMB WITH CARAMELISED SHALLOTS

SERVES 6
PER SERVING 355 KCAL/21G FAT

900g (2lb) lamb fillet
24 button shallots, peeled
24 button mushrooms
24 pomodorino tomatoes or cherry tomatoes
1 teaspoon sugar
1 tablespoon balsamic vinegar
1 tablespoon chopped flat leaf parsley
sea salt and freshly ground black pepper

for the marinade
1 tablespoon finely chopped fresh rosemary
1 red onion, finely chopped
2 garlic cloves, chopped
3 tablespoons mint jelly
1 teaspoon coarsely ground black pepper
1 wineglass white wine

Combine all the marinade ingredients in a bowl.

Prepare the meat by removing all visible fat with a sharp knife. Place the meat in a shallow dish and pour the marinade over the meat. Turn the meat so that all sides are coated with the marinade. Cover with food wrap and chill for at least 4 hours.

Thirty minutes before cooking, remove the lamb from the marinade and place on a grill tray. Pour the marinade into a small saucepan and reduce it over a low heat for 10 minutes.

Preheat the grill to the hottest setting. Season the lamb all over with salt and black pepper and place under the hot grill. Cook for 15–20 minutes, turning regularly. Allow to stand for 10 minutes before carving.

While the lamb is cooking, preheat a non-stick frying pan. Add the shallots and the sugar and cook over a high heat for 5–6 minutes until golden. Add the mushrooms and season well with salt and black pepper.

Just before serving, add the tomatoes, balsamic vinegar and parsley. Mix well.

To serve, carve the lamb into small chunky slices. Place on top of the vegetables and drizzle the marinade over.

ORIENTAL PAN-COOKED PORK

SERVES 2
PER SERVING 270 KCAL/7.8G FAT

4 tablespoons Sharwoods plum sauce
1 teaspoon soy sauce
225g (8oz) lean pork tenderloin, thinly sliced
2 garlic cloves, crushed
1 red chilli, finely sliced
1 celery stick, cut into strips
115g (4oz) pak choi, shredded or quartered lengthways if
small, or 115g (4oz) Chinese leaf, shredded
4 spring onions, sliced
salt and freshly ground black pepper

Mix together the plum and soy sauce in a bowl.

Dry-fry the pork, garlic and chilli in a large non-stick wok or saucepan for 3–4 minutes or until browned. Add the celery and cook for a further 1–2 minutes. Add the remaining ingredients and cook for 1–2 minutes.

Drizzle with the plum and soy sauce and serve immediately.

RANCHERO PIE

SERVES 4
PER SERVING 495 KCAL/13.6G FAT

450g (1lb) lean pork mince
1 onion, chopped
1 × 400g (14oz) tin mixed beans in chilli sauce
4 tablespoons tomato passata
1 tablespoon mild chilli sauce or 1 teaspoon chilli powder
1 tablespoon chopped fresh mixed herbs (e.g. chives,
oregano, parsley)

for the topping
675g (1½lb) potatoes, peeled and chopped
1 × 200g (7oz) tin sweetcorn, drained
2 tablespoons skimmed milk
1 tablespoon chopped fresh parsley
25g (1oz) grated low-fat cheese

Preheat the oven to 190C, 375F, Gas Mark 5. To make
the topping, boil the potatoes until softened, then drain
them. Mash the potatoes with the sweetcorn, milk and
parsley.

Meanwhile, in a large non-stick saucepan, dry-fry
the mince and onion for about 4–6 minutes, until they
change colour. Add the beans, passata and chilli sauce
or powder, bring to the boil and simmer for 3–5 minutes.
Transfer the mixture to an ovenproof dish. Top with the
mashed potato, and sprinkle with the cheese. Bake in
the oven for 20 minutes.

PORK AND APPLE BURGERS IN PITTA BREAD

SERVES 4
PER SERVING 296 KCAL/8.5G FAT

350g (12oz) lean pork mince
6 tablespoons unsweetened apple sauce
50g (2oz) fresh brown breadcrumbs
1 teaspoon dried sage
175g (6oz) mushrooms, sliced
a little vegetable stock
4 tomatoes, halved
4 small wholemeal pitta breads
salt and freshly ground black pepper

Place the pork, apple sauce, breadcrumbs and sage in a mixing bowl. Season with salt and pepper and mix until well combined. With well-floured hands, form the pork mixture into 4 burger shapes. Cover and chill until required.

Cook under a preheated grill for about 8–10 minutes each side, turning once.

Meanwhile, place the mushrooms in a small pan and add just enough stock to cover them. Bring to the boil then simmer gently for 2–3 minutes until the mushrooms are tender. Cook the tomatoes under the grill for about 5 minutes. Lightly toast the pitta breads if desired.

Serve the burgers with the pitta breads, tomatoes and mushrooms.

GAMMON WITH PINEAPPLE RICE

SERVES 1
PER SERVING 431 KCAL/5.5G FAT

1 gammon steak
1 small onion, finely chopped
1 small tin pineapple chunks in natural juice
$\frac{1}{2}$ vegetable stock cube
50g (2oz) [dry weight] brown rice
50g (2oz) tinned or frozen peas
$\frac{1}{2}$ red pepper, sliced
dash of soy sauce
1 tablespoon chopped fresh chives
salt and freshly ground black pepper

Cut the gammon steak into cubes and gently dry-fry with the onion in a non-stick pan. Add the pineapple and juice, the stock cube, rice and approximately 300ml ($\frac{1}{2}$ pint) water and bring to the boil. Cover and cook for 10 minutes or until the rice is tender and most of the liquid is absorbed. Add more boiling water during cooking if necessary.

Stir in the peas, red pepper and soy sauce and season to taste. Finally, stir in the chives, heat through and serve immediately.

PORK AND MANGO MEATBALLS WITH CHILLI SAUCE

SERVES 4
PER SERVING 255 KCAL/11.5G FAT

450g (1lb) lean minced pork
1 medium onion, finely chopped
1 teaspoon ground cumin
1 teaspoon ground coriander
1 tablespoon chopped fresh parsley
1 teaspoon salt
freshly ground black pepper
2 tablespoons spicy mango chutney

for the sauce
1 x 400g (14oz) tin chopped tomatoes
1 small red chilli, seeded and finely chopped
1 vegetable stock cube
2 tablespoons tomato purée
1 tablespoon chopped fresh coriander

Preheat the oven to 200C, 400F, Gas Mark 6. In a large mixing bowl combine the pork with the other ingredients, mixing well with a wooden spoon. Season with black pepper.

Form the mixture into golf ball size pieces, roll until smooth and place in an ovenproof dish.

Combine the sauce ingredients together in a saucepan and bring to the boil. Pour over the meat balls and place in the oven for 35–40 minutes.

GINGERED PORK WITH APRICOTS

SERVES 4
PER SERVING 265 KCAL/7.5G FAT

450g (1lb) lean pork, cubed
1 medium onion, chopped
1 teaspoon dried ginger
1 teaspoon chopped fresh thyme
75g (3oz) ready-to-use dried apricots
600ml (1 pint) stock
salt and freshly ground black pepper
2 teaspoons cornflour

Preheat the oven to 180C, 350F, Gas Mark 4. Dry-fry the pork and onion in a hot, heavy-based pan until the pork is browned. Add the ginger, thyme, apricots and stock. Season to taste with salt and pepper and bring to the boil.

Mix the cornflour with a little water and stir into the pan, mixing well.

Pour the meat and sauce into a casserole dish. Cover and place in the oven for 1–1¼ hours until the pork is tender.

THAI CHICKEN

SERVES 4
PER SERVING 204 KCAL/7.4G FAT

4 skinned chicken breasts
1 red pepper, finely sliced
6 spring onions, finely chopped
6 plum tomatoes skinned, seeded and diced
1 green chilli, seeded and finely chopped
zest and juice of 2 limes
2 garlic cloves, crushed
1 teaspoon ground cumin
1 teaspoon ground coriander
1 tablespoon cornflour
300ml ($\frac{1}{2}$ pint) pineapple juice
salt and freshly ground black pepper
chopped fresh coriander to garnish

Preheat the oven to 190C, 375F, Gas Mark 5. Place the chicken in an ovenproof dish and season well on both sides with salt and pepper.

Place the red pepper, onions and tomatoes in a bowl. Add the chilli, lime juice and zest, garlic, cumin and coriander and combine well.

Dissolve the cornflour with the pineapple juice and pour over the vegetables. Mix well and season with plenty of salt and pepper. Pour over the chicken and bake in the oven for 30–35 minutes. Garnish with coriander and serve immediately.

TARRAGON CHICKEN WITH MUSHROOM SAUCE

SERVES 2
PER SERVING 376 KCAL/11.8G FAT

1 onion, finely chopped
115g (4oz) chestnut mushrooms, finely chopped
1 tablespoon chopped fresh tarragon
4 skinless chicken breasts
300ml (½ pint) skimmed milk
1 tablespoon coarse grain mustard
1 tablespoon cornflour
salt and freshly ground black pepper

In a non-stick frying pan, dry-fry the onion and the mushrooms for 2–3 minutes, seasoning with salt and pepper. Add the tarragon and mix well. Remove from the heat.

Preheat the oven to 200C, 400F, Gas Mark 6. Place the chicken breasts on a board. Using a sharp knife, make an incision halfway up the side to create a pocket. Place a tablespoonful of onion and mushroom mixture inside each chicken breast and arrange in the bottom of an ovenproof dish. Season with salt and black pepper.

Return the frying pan containing the remaining mixture to the stove, and add the skimmed milk and mustard.

Mix the cornflour with a little cold water and stir into the sauce. Continue stirring and bring to the boil, allowing the sauce to thicken. Pour the sauce over the chicken breasts and cover with aluminium foil. Place in the oven for 30–35 minutes.

STICKY GINGER CHICKEN

SERVES 2
PER SERVING 308 KCAL/7.6G FAT

2 tablespoons lemon juice
2 tablespoons light Muscovado sugar
1 teaspoon grated fresh ginger
2 teaspoons soy sauce
8 chicken drumsticks or thighs
freshly ground black pepper
salt to taste (optional)

In a mixing bowl, mix together the lemon juice, sugar, ginger, soy sauce and pepper to form a glaze. Taste, and add a little salt if wished.

Remove the skin and any fat from the drumsticks or thighs. Slash the flesh on each one 2 or 3 times and toss the chicken in the glaze.

Cook the chicken under a moderately hot grill, turning them occasionally and brushing with the glaze. Cook until the juices run clear when the flesh is pierced with a skewer.

CHICKEN LIVER STROGANOFF

SERVES 4
PER SERVING 175 KCAL/3.6G FAT

450g (1lb) chicken livers
1 medium onion, finely chopped
2 garlic cloves, crushed
1 tablespoon plain flour
2 tablespoons Madeira wine
150ml (1/4 pint) chicken stock
225g (8oz) small chestnut mushrooms, sliced
2 teaspoons Dijon mustard
300ml (1/2 pint) virtually fat free fromage frais
2 tablespoons chopped fresh parsley
salt and freshly ground black pepper
lemon wedges and paprika to garnish

Check the chicken livers and remove any sinews or fat. Rinse well in clean water and leave to dry on kitchen paper.

Preheat a non-stick frying pan or wok. Dry-fry the onion for 2–3 minutes until soft. Add the garlic and cook for a further minute. Toss the chicken livers in the flour, season well with salt and black pepper and add to the pan. Cook quickly over a high heat for 1 minute. Add the Madeira wine and gradually the stock to form a thick sauce. Add the mushrooms, stir in the mustard and cook for a further minute. The chicken livers should be firm but not overcooked.

Remove the pan from the heat and stir in the fromage frais and parsley. Check the seasoning. Garnish with lemon wedges and dust with paprika. Serve immediately.

BASIL CHICKEN

SERVES 4
PER SERVING 251 KCAL/6.8G FAT

4 x 115g (4×4oz) boned and skinned chicken breasts
chopped fresh basil to taste
4 tablespoons fresh white breadcrumbs
salt and freshly ground black pepper
a little skimmed milk
175–225g (6–8oz) fresh asparagus spears or
1×400g (14oz) tin asparagus spears to
garnish (optional)

Preheat the oven to 180C, 350F, Gas Mark 4. Slightly flatten the chicken breasts.

Add plenty of basil to the breadcrumbs so that the mixture smells strongly of the herb. Season with salt and lots of black pepper.

Dip the chicken breasts into the milk and coat with the breadcrumb and herb mixture.

Dry-fry the chicken in a non-stick pan for a few minutes until both sides are brown. Place the chicken breasts on a non-stick baking tray and cook in the oven for 15 minutes. Just before serving, garnish with asparagus spears (if using).

CHICKEN CURRY

SERVES 2
PER SERVING 229 KCAL/6G FAT

2 chicken breasts, all fat and skin removed
1 × 400g (14oz) tin tomatoes
1 bay leaf
1 eating apple, cored and chopped small
2 teaspoons Branston pickle
1 teaspoon tomato purée
1 medium onion, finely chopped
1 tablespoon curry powder

Place the chicken breasts and the remaining ingredients in a saucepan and bring to the boil. Place a lid on the saucepan and cook slowly for about 1 hour, stirring occasionally, and turning the chicken breasts every 15 minutes or so. If the sauce is too thin, remove the lid and cook on a slightly higher heat until the sauce reduces and thickens. Remove bay leaf before serving.

TURKEY CHILLI PASTA

SERVES 2
PER SERVING 494 KCAL/3.6G FAT

350g (12oz) turkey mince
1 medium onion, chopped
2 garlic cloves, crushed
1 red chilli, seeded and finely chopped
1 × 400g (14oz) tin chopped tomatoes

2 teaspoons freeze-dried fines herbes
2 tablespoons tomato purée
300ml (1/2 pint) chicken stock
175g (6oz) [dry weight] pasta shells
salt and freshly ground black pepper
1 tablespoon chopped fresh parsley

In a large non-stick saucepan, dry-fry the turkey mince with the onion and until the mince changes colour and forms a firm consistency. Add the remaining ingredients and simmer for 20–25 minutes until the pasta is cooked.

LEMON ROAST TURKEY WITH CORNBREAD STUFFING AND HERB GRAVY

SERVES 8–10
PER SERVING 302 KCAL/3.5G FAT

1 × 5.4kg (12lb) fresh turkey
1 large onion, diced
3 bay leaves
4–5 sprigs fresh thyme
3 lemons
pinch of sea salt
1 teaspoon lemon pepper
1 tablespoon arrowroot
few drops of gravy browning (optional)

for the stuffing
175g (6oz) plain flour
175g (6oz) fine cornmeal

1 tablespoon baking powder
1 teaspoon salt
1 tablespoon caster sugar
2 tablespoons chopped fresh mixed herbs (oregano,
thyme, marjoram, parsley)
1 egg, beaten
300ml (½ pint) skimmed milk

Preheat the oven to 180C, 350F, Gas Mark 4. Wash the turkey in cold water, remove the giblets and any fat. Place the giblets, onion, bay leaves and 2 sprigs of thyme in the centre of a large roasting tin and sit the turkey on top.

Cut the lemons in half and squeeze the juice from all three over the turkey. Place the lemon shells and the remaining thyme inside the turkey. Season the turkey with sea salt and lemon pepper. Pour 600ml (1 pint) of water around the outside of the turkey to prevent the base from burning, cover with aluminium foil and place in the oven. Cook for the recommended time (allow 15 minutes per 450g/lb, plus an extra 20 minutes), turning the roasting tin every hour to ensure even cooking.

Once the turkey is cooked, remove from the tin and place on a serving dish. Keep it covered with foil and allow 30 minutes' standing time for easier carving.

Increase the oven temperature to 200C, 400F, Gas Mark 6. Lightly grease and line a 20cm (8in) cake tin with baking parchment. To make the cornbread stuffing, mix together the dry ingredients and herbs in a large bowl. Beat together the egg and milk and add to the dry ingredients. Mix until smooth, then pour into the prepared tin. Bake in the oven for 25–35 minutes until golden brown.

Meanwhile, drain the contents of the roasting tin into a saucepan. Remove the giblets and bay leaves and discard. Use a ladle to skim away any fat from the top of the pan. Bring the liquid to the boil, slake the arrowroot with a little water and gradually add to the gravy, stirring well. Add a few drops of gravy browning, if desired, to colour the gravy. Thin down with vegetable stock if required.

To serve, carve the turkey and serve with the corn-bread stuffing and herb gravy.

Fish

FISHERMAN'S PIE

SERVES 6
PER SERVING 258 KCAL/2G FAT

675g (1½lb) potatoes, peeled
2 tablespoons low-fat natural yogurt
350g (12oz) smoked haddock
350g (12oz) cod or white haddock
225g (8oz) peeled and cooked prawns
2 baby leeks, chopped
150ml (¼ pint) fish stock
1 tablespoon flour
½ wineglass white wine
1 tablespoon Dijon mustard
600ml (1 pint) skimmed milk
2 tablespoons capers
salt and freshly ground black pepper
chopped fresh parsley to garnish

Preheat the oven to 220C, 425F, Gas Mark 7. Boil the potatoes in a saucepan of water until well done. Drain and mash until smooth. Mix in the yogurt and season well with salt and black pepper.

Remove the skin and bones from the fish. Cut into bite-sized pieces and place in the bottom of an oven-proof dish. Add the prawns.

Place the leeks and the fish stock in a medium saucepan and cook for 1–2 minutes. Sprinkle the flour over and mix well. Cook for a further minute in order to cook out the flour. Add the wine and mustard and beat well. Gradually add the skimmed milk, stirring continuously to prevent any lumps from forming. Bring to the boil, allowing the sauce to thicken. Pour over the fish and sprinkle the capers on top. Allow to cool for 20 minutes, then cover with the mashed potato, either using a fork or piping through a piping bag with a large star nozzle.

Place in the oven for 30–40 minutes until golden.

Just before serving, sprinkle with the chopped parsley.

SMOKED HADDOCK FISH CAKES WITH CAPER SAUCE

SERVES 4
PER SERVING 242 KCAL/1.7G FAT

450g (1lb) fresh smoked haddock
450g (1lb) cooked mashed potato
2 baby leeks, finely chopped
zest and juice of 1 lemon

2 tablespoons chopped fresh parsley
1 teaspoon coarse grain mustard
salt and freshly ground black pepper

for the caper sauce
175g (6oz) virtually fat free fromage frais
1 tablespoon cider vinegar
1 tablespoon lemon juice
$\frac{1}{4}$ teaspoon ground turmeric
2 teaspoons sugar
1 tablespoon chopped fresh parsley
1 tablespoon chopped capers
salt and freshly ground black pepper

Poach the smoked haddock in a little water until just cooked. Remove from the pan with a slotted spoon and allow to cool. Place the mashed potato in a large bowl. Flake the fish into the bowl, removing any skin and bones.

In a non-stick frying pan, dry-fry the leeks until soft. Add to the potato mixture, then add the lemon zest and juice, parsley and mustard. Mix well and season with plenty of salt and black pepper.

Shape the mixture into 8 small balls, then gently flatten with a palette knife to form fish cakes. Dry-fry in a non-stick pan on both sides until golden brown then transfer to the oven to keep warm.

Combine all the sauce ingredients in a bowl.

Serve the fish cakes hot with the caper sauce.

PAN-FRIED TUNA WITH PEPPER NOODLES

SERVES 4

PER SERVING 356 KCAL/8.6G FAT

4 fresh tuna steaks
225g (8oz) [dry weight] thread noodles
1 teaspoon vegetable oil
1 garlic clove, crushed
1 red pepper, seeded and finely sliced
1 yellow pepper, seeded and finely sliced
zest and juice of 1 lime
1 tablespoon light soy sauce
salt and freshly ground black pepper
4 lime slices and red pepper to garnish

Trim the tuna steaks with a sharp knife, removing any unsightly dark fish. Season well with salt and black pepper.

Prepare the noodles by placing in boiling salted water for 2–3 minutes. Drain and refresh under cold running water.

Heat a griddle pan or non-stick frying pan, add the vegetable oil and then wipe out the pan with a piece of kitchen paper, taking care not to burn your fingers (use an oven glove if necessary).

Place the tuna, best side down, in the hot pan. As the tuna cooks it will change colour. Rather like a thermometer, the colour band will change and move up the fish. When it reaches halfway up the steaks, turn the steaks over and cook for a few minutes. Remove from the pan and place in a warm oven to keep hot.

Add the garlic and peppers to the pan and sauté quickly until they start to soften. Add the noodles, lime zest and juice and soy sauce. Cook for 1–2 minutes, turning regularly. Place the noodles on warmed serving plates and top with the tuna steak. Garnish each one with a slice of lime and red pepper.

SPICY KING PRAWNS

SERVES 2
PER SERVING 116 KCAL/1G FAT

1 medium onion, finely diced
2 garlic cloves, crushed
1 red pepper, seeded and finely diced
20 medium uncooked king prawns, peeled
2 × 400g (2 × 14oz) tins chopped tomatoes
2 teaspoons chilli sauce
1 teaspoon lemon grass
1 tablespoon bouillon stock powder
2 tablespoons chopped fresh parsley
salt and freshly ground black pepper
1 teaspoon finely chopped lemon grass

Dry-fry the onion and garlic in a non-stick frying pan. Add the red pepper and cook for a further minute. Add the prawns and quickly seal (do not overcook). Cover with the tomatoes. Add the chilli sauce, lemon grass and the bouillon stock powder. Bring the sauce to the boil, and simmer for 1–2 minutes until the prawns are cooked through. Season well with salt and black pepper.

Just before serving, sprinkle with the parsley.

SMOKED HAM AND PRAWN JAMBALYA

SERVES 4
PER SERVING 225 KCAL/3.1G FAT

2 medium onions, chopped
2 garlic cloves, crushed
2 celery sticks, diced
1 × 400g (14oz) tin chopped tomatoes
2 tablespoons tomato purée
1 red chilli, seeded and finely chopped
225g (8oz) cooked long grain rice
225g (8oz) smoked ham, cut into bite-sized pieces
225g (8oz) peeled and cooked prawns
1 tablespoon chopped fresh mixed herbs
(e.g. chives, parsley and tarragon)
freshly grated nutmeg
salt and freshly ground black pepper

Dry-fry the onion and garlic in a non-stick pan until soft. Add the celery, tomatoes, tomato purée and chilli and simmer for 10 minutes. Add the rice, smoked ham, prawns, grated nutmeg and herbs and simmer for a further 2–3 minutes, making sure the ham and prawns are heated through. Season to taste.

SEAFOOD KEDGEREE

SERVES 4

PER SERVING 339 KCAL/3G FAT

1 large onion, finely chopped
225g (8oz) long grain rice
1 teaspoon mild curry powder
450ml (¾ pint) vegetable stock
1 small red chilli, finely sliced
2 bay leaves
450g (1lb) cooked seafood (e.g. mussels,
prawns, crab, squid, smoked fish)
salt and freshly ground black pepper

In a non-stick saucepan, dry-fry the onion for 2–3 minutes until soft. Add the rice and curry powder, and gradually stir in the stock. Add the chilli and bay leaves, bring to the boil, reduce the heat and place a lid on the pan. Simmer, covered, for 20 minutes until most of the liquid has been absorbed.

Add the seafood, season to taste and heat through for 5 minutes to ensure that the seafood is hot, adding a little stock if required. Remove bay leaves before serving.

ROASTED MONKFISH CHERMOULA

SERVES 4

PER SERVING 234 KCAL/2.8G FAT

900g (2lb) monkfish tail fillets, cut into 4 pieces
1 medium red onion, finely diced

1 teaspoon ground cumin
1 teaspoon ground paprika
1 teaspoon ground turmeric
good pinch of saffron
1 small red chilli, seeded and finely chopped
zest and juice of 1 lemon
3 tablespoons fresh orange juice
6 tablespoons chopped fresh coriander
900g (2lb) pousse (baby spinach)
pinch of ground cinnamon
salt and freshly ground black pepper

Prepare the monkfish by removing the thin outer skin and any bones. Rinse well and place the pieces side by side in a large ovenproof dish. Sprinkle the red onion over the top and season well with salt and black pepper.

In a small bowl combine the spices with the chilli, lemon zest and juice and the orange juice. Spoon the marinade over the fish, then turn the fillets to coat all sides with the spices. Cover and place in refrigerator for 30 minutes to allow the spices to penetrate.

Preheat the oven to 190C, 375F, Gas Mark 5. When the fish has marinated, transfer to a non-stick roasting tin, pour the marinade over the fish and sprinkle with coriander. Place in the oven for 12–15 minutes until just cooked.

Wash the spinach and place in a preheated non-stick wok. Season well with salt and black pepper, add a pinch of cinnamon and cook over a high heat for 1–2 minutes, stirring well.

Serve the monkfish on a bed of spinach and pour the juices over the top.

Vegetarian

LEEK AND SUN-DRIED TOMATO RISOTTO CAKES

SERVES 4
PER SERVING 262 KCAL/3.6G FAT

1 large onion, finely chopped
2 garlic cloves, crushed
225g (8oz) [dry weight] risotto rice
600ml (1 pint) vegetable stock
2 leeks, finely chopped
4 sun-dried tomatoes, finely chopped
1 tablespoon chopped fresh chervil
2 tablespoons plain flour
salt and freshly ground black pepper

In a non-stick pan dry-fry the onion and garlic until soft. Add the rice, and gradually stir in the stock a little at a time until most of the stock has been absorbed. Stir in the chopped leeks, tomatoes, chervil and remaining stock. Season with salt and pepper and allow to cool.

Mould the risotto mixture into fish-cake shapes, allowing 1 large or 2 small cakes per person. Use the flour to prevent them from sticking to your hands. Shape with a palette knife.

Preheat a non-stick frying pan. Dry-fry the risotto cakes for 2–3 minutes on each side until lightly golden. Serve hot.

SPICY CHICKPEA CASSEROLE

SERVES 4
PER SERVING 426 KCAL/5.7G FAT

225g (8oz) [dry weight] chickpeas, soaked overnight
1 medium onion, chopped
1 × 400g (14oz) tin chopped tomatoes
2 vegetable stock cubes
$\frac{1}{2}$ teaspoon ground coriander
2 heaped teaspoons cumin seeds
$\frac{1}{2}$ teaspoon chilli powder
225g (8oz) [dry weight] brown rice
225g (8oz) mushrooms, sliced
1 tablespoon chopped fresh coriander
salt and freshly ground black pepper

Fast-boil the chickpeas for 10 minutes, then simmer for a further 20–25 minutes until fairly soft. Meanwhile, place the onion and tomatoes into a medium saucepan with one of the stock cubes. Add the coriander, cumin, chilli and season with salt and black pepper. Bring to the boil and simmer gently for 10 minutes.

Cook the rice according to the packet instructions, adding the remaining vegetable stock cube to the cooking water. Drain well and keep hot.

When the chickpeas are almost cooked, drain them, then rinse with boiling water. Stir the chickpeas into the tomato and spice mixture. Add the mushrooms and simmer for a further 5 minutes. Season well with salt and black pepper, add the fresh coriander and serve with the rice and a salad.

BEAN AND BURGUNDY CASSEROLE

SERVES 6
PER SERVING 326 KCAL/4G FAT

175g (6oz) [dry weight] green lentils
1 tablespoon vegetable oil
2 medium onions, finely chopped
2 garlic cloves, crushed
2 teaspoons cumin seeds
1 teaspoon dried oregano
300ml (½ pint) red wine
1 × 400g (14oz) tin chopped tomatoes
450–600ml (¾–1 pint) vegetable stock
1 bay leaf
450g (1lb) firm old or new potatoes, peeled and
cut into large dice
1–2 large carrots, sliced
225g (8oz) leeks, cut into 2.5cm (1in) lengths
1 × 400g (14oz) tin red kidney beans, drained and rinsed
175–225g (6–8oz) small button mushrooms
1 small cauliflower, broken into florets (optional)
salt and freshly ground black pepper
1 tablespoon chopped fresh parsley to garnish

Soak the lentils in cold water for at least an hour. Drain.

Heat the oil in a large pan and cook the onions gently until soft. Add the garlic, cumin seeds and oregano and cook for a further 2–3 minutes. Add the drained lentils, wine, tomatoes, 450ml (¾ pint) of the vegetable stock and the bay leaf. Bring to the boil, cover the pan and simmer for 10–15 minutes.

Add the potatoes, carrots, leeks and kidney beans to the pan. Bring back to the boil again, adding more stock if necessary, and simmer for a further 10 minutes.

Add the mushrooms and cauliflower (if using) to the pan and continue cooking for a further 7–10 minutes or until the lentils are tender.

When the lentils are tender, remove the bay leaf from the pan and season the vegetables to taste with salt and pepper. Just before serving, pour the casserole into a hot serving dish and sprinkle the chopped parsley over the top.

STIR-FRY QUORN

SERVES 4
PER SERVING 130 KCAL/4.8G FAT

1 teaspoon sunflower oil
450g (16oz) Quorn chunks
2 teaspoons ground coriander
8 spring onions, chopped
115g (4oz) pak choi or spring greens
115g (4oz) mange tout
2 medium carrots, cut into julienne strips
grated root ginger to taste
1–2 teaspoons soy sauce
juice of 1 lemon
salt and freshly ground black pepper

Heat the oil in a wok or non-stick pan. Add the Quorn, ground coriander and spring onions and cook for a few minutes.

Add the remaining vegetables and the grated ginger. Continue to cook until the Quorn and vegetables are cooked but the vegetables are still crunchy. Add the soy sauce and lemon juice. Season to taste and serve immediately.

LENTIL AND POTATO PIE

SERVES 3
PER SERVING 339 KCAL/1.2G FAT

175g (6oz) red lentils
1 large onion, chopped
350g (12oz) potatoes, peeled
2 tablespoons pickle
1 teaspoon mixed herbs
salt and freshly ground black pepper
paprika

Rinse the lentils. Place the lentils and onion in a pan, cover with water and cook slowly for about 20 minutes until the lentils are tender and all the water is absorbed.

Preheat the oven to 200C, 400F, Gas Mark 6. Cook the potatoes in boiling salted water. When cooked, drain well and mash. Beat the mashed potato into the lentils. Add the pickle, herbs and plenty of salt and pepper and mix well.

Place the mixture in a shallow ovenproof dish. Fork the top and sprinkle a little paprika over it. Bake in the oven for 20 minutes until crisp and brown.

ADUKI BEAN PIE WITH POTATO AND CHIVE TOPPING

SERVES 4
PER SERVING 468 KCAL/3.4G FAT

350g (12oz) dry Aduki beans (soaked overnight)
2 onions, finely chopped
2 celery sticks, finely chopped
1 vegetable stock cube
1 × 400g (14oz) tin chopped tomatoes
600ml (1 pint) tomato passata
1 tablespoon chopped fresh mixed herbs

for the topping
900g (2lb) boiling potatoes
3 tablespoons low-fat natural yogurt
2 tablespoons chopped fresh chives
salt and freshly ground black pepper

Drain the Aduki beans and rinse well with fresh water. Place in a saucepan and cover with water. Bring to the boil and simmer for 30 minutes until tender.

Meanwhile, in a non-stick frying pan, dry-fry the onions and celery until soft, add the remaining ingredients and simmer for 10 minutes.

Preheat the oven to 200C, 400F, Gas Mark 6. Boil the potatoes until cooked, drain well and mash until smooth. Season well with salt and black pepper, mix in the yogurt and chives. Drain the Aduki beans and add to the sauce. Pour into an ovenproof dish and top with the potatoes. Place in the oven for 20 minutes or until golden brown. Serve hot.

AUBERGINE TAGINE WITH ROAST GARLIC

SERVES 2
PER SERVING 206 KCAL/3G FAT

3 medium aubergines
4 garlic cloves, peeled
small bulb of fennel
2 medium red onions
2 red peppers, seeded
1 teaspoon ground cumin
$\frac{1}{2}$ teaspoon ground cinnamon
1 teaspoon ground coriander
1 × 400g (14oz) tin chopped tomatoes
150ml ($\frac{1}{4}$ pint) vegetable stock
1 orange
6 cardamom pods
2 tablespoons tomato purée
2 tablespoons finely chopped fresh flat leaf parsley
salt and freshly ground black pepper
extra chopped fresh flat leaf parsley to garnish

Preheat the oven to 200C, 400F, Gas Mark 6. Take 2 of the aubergines and slice down the centre lengthways with a sharp knife. Using a dessertspoon, scoop out the centres, taking care not to damage the outer skin. Season the shells with salt and black pepper and place, skin-side up, on a baking sheet. Bake in the oven for 20–25 minutes until soft. Remove and set aside. While the aubergines are baking, wrap 4 garlic cloves in a small piece of aluminium foil and place in the oven for 20 minutes.

Prepare the fennel and the remaining vegetables by cutting into rough pieces, about 1cm (½in) thick. Preheat a large non-stick saucepan, add the vegetables and cook briskly for 8–10 minutes, stirring occasionally, until they start to brown. Add the spices and roast garlic and cook for 1 minute before adding the chopped tomatoes and stock.

Using a vegetable peeler, remove 3 strips of orange peel from the orange, and then squeeze out the juice from the orange. Add the strips of orange peel and the orange juice to the pan.

Place the cardamom pods on a chopping board. Using the broad blade of a chopping knife, crush the pods and remove the inner black seeds. Discard the pods and crush the black seeds, then add the seeds, tomato purée and parsley to the pan. Reduce the heat and simmer gently for 20 minutes until the sauce thickens. Place the pre-roasted aubergine shells into an ovenproof dish, spoon in the tagine and bake in the preheated oven for 10–15 minutes.

Just before serving, garnish with chopped fresh flat leaf parsley. Serve hot.

MINTED SAFFRON COUSCOUS

SERVES 2
PER SERVING 236 KCAL/2G FAT

400ml (14fl oz) vegetable stock
1/4 teaspoon ground cumin
1/4 teaspoon paprika
1/4 teaspoon ground coriander
good pinch of saffron
175g (6oz) [dry weight] couscous
4 tomatoes
salt and freshly ground black pepper
juice of 1/2 lemon
2 tablespoons chopped fresh mint to garnish

In a saucepan bring the stock to the boil, add the spices and then the couscous, stir well, and cover with a lid for 1 minute.

Blanch the tomatoes in boiling water for just 10 seconds and then immediately submerge in cold water and remove the skins.

Remove the lid from the couscous and fluff up the couscous, using a fork to separate the grains, then cover again.

Cut the tomatoes in half. Place them in the cold water to remove the seeds, then rinse the tomatoes. Chop into small dice and add to the couscous, along with the chopped mint.

Season with salt and black pepper and spoon into a warmed serving dish. Drizzle with lemon juice and garnish with fresh mint.

VEGETARIAN LOAF

SERVES 4
PER SERVING 238 KCAL/11.8G FAT

450g (1lb) medium tofu
250ml (8fl oz) bolognese sauce (low-fat
vegetarian brand)
1 medium onion, chopped
1 green pepper, seeded and chopped
1 garlic clove, crushed
1 teaspoon dried oregano
$\frac{1}{2}$ teaspoon dried basil
25g (1oz) oats
25g (1oz) wholemeal flour
salt and freshly ground black pepper

Preheat the oven to 180C, 350F, Gas Mark 4. Very lightly oil a 10 × 20cm (4 × 8in) baking tin.

Rinse and drain the tofu and place it in a large bowl with half the bolognese sauce. Add the chopped onion, green pepper, garlic and herbs and mash well with a fork. Add the oats and the wholemeal flour, season with salt and pepper to taste and mix well. Press the mixture into the prepared tin and press down firmly. Bake in the oven for 45 minutes.

Heat the remaining sauce. Remove the loaf from the oven and allow to stand for 5 minutes before inverting onto a serving dish. Serve with the hot sauce.

BUTTERNUT SQUASH AND LEEK RISOTTO WITH SUN-DRIED TOMATOES

SERVES 4

PER SERVING 275 KCAL/3.4G FAT

2 medium butternut squash
1 medium onion, finely chopped
225g (8oz) [dry weight] risotto rice
900ml (1½ pints) vegetable stock
2 leeks, finely chopped
4 sun-dried tomatoes (non-oil variety), finely chopped
1 tablespoon chopped fresh chervil
salt and freshly ground black pepper
4 parsley sprigs to garnish

Preheat the oven to 220C, 425F, Gas Mark 7. Slice both squash lengthways and scoop out the seeds with a spoon. Carefully scoop out some of the flesh, taking care not to break the outer skin. Dice the flesh and set aside.

Season the squash shells and place the 4 halves face-down in an ovenproof dish. Bake in the oven for 15–20 minutes until tender.

While the squash are baking, start to make the risotto by dry-frying the onion and squash flesh in a non-stick frying pan until soft. Add the rice and the vegetable stock. Bring to the boil, add the leek and tomatoes, cover with a lid and reduce the heat to a low setting. Simmer gently, stirring occasionally, for 20 minutes or until all the stock has been absorbed and rice is cooked.

Add the chervil to the risotto and adjust the seasoning to taste. Spoon the risotto into the squash shells, garnish with the parsley sprigs and serve immediately.

AUBERGINE AND GINGER PARCELS

SERVES 2
PER SERVING 398 KCAL/15.4G FAT

1 medium aubergine
1 medium onion, finely chopped
2 garlic cloves, crushed
1 tablespoon finely chopped fresh ginger
300ml ($\frac{1}{2}$ pint) tomato passata
1 vegetable stock cube
1 tablespoon chopped fresh parsley
1 egg
3 tablespoons skimmed milk
8 sheets filo pastry
1 tablespoon sesame seeds
salt and black pepper

Prepare the aubergine by slicing off the hard stem at the top. Using a chopping knife, cut thick slices from the length of the aubergine. Cut these slices into strips and then into small dice. Season well with salt and black pepper.

Preheat a non-stick frying pan, add the onion and dry-fry until soft. Add the diced aubergine and crushed garlic and cook for 3–4 minutes. Stir in the ginger, passata, stock cube and parsley. Season with salt and pepper. Simmer for 10 minutes until the liquid has reduced to leave a thick chunky paste. Allow to cool.

Preheat the oven to 220C, 425F, Gas Mark 7. Beat together the egg and milk. Take one sheet of filo pastry and brush with the egg and milk mixture. Fold a third of the long side into the centre and again on the other side to leave a long, thin strip of pastry. Brush again with the egg and milk. Place a good tablespoon of mixture at one end of the pastry and fold over diagonally, enclosing the mixture in a triangle. Fold the pastry back over along the length of the pastry, retaining the triangle shape and tucking in any spare ends.

Brush with the egg and milk, place on a baking tray and sprinkle with the sesame seeds. Repeat this process for all 8 parcels.

Bake in the oven for 20–25 minutes until golden brown.

VEGETABLE CRUNCH

SERVES 2
PER SERVING 364 KCAL/3G FAT

1 medium onion, roughly chopped

1 leek, sliced

1 celery stick, chopped

175g (6oz) mushrooms, sliced

450g (1lb) potatoes, peeled and cut into large pieces

175g (6oz) carrots, sliced

1/2 small cauliflower, broken into small florets

1 tablespoon stuffing mix

for the sauce
300ml (½ pint) skimmed milk
2 teaspoons cornflour
salt and black pepper to taste
2 tablespoons chopped fresh parsley

Dry-fry the onion, leek, celery and mushrooms for 3–5 minutes until soft.

Place the potatoes in a large saucepan, cover with cold water and bring to the boil. Add the carrots and cook for 5 minutes. Add the cauliflower and gently boil until all the vegetables are just cooked. Drain and reserve the vegetable water.

Preheat the oven to 180C, 350F, Gas Mark 4.

To make the sauce, reserve 2 tablespoons of the milk and heat the rest in a saucepan. Mix the reserved milk with the cornflour. Gradually whisk in the hot milk and 150ml (¼ pint) of the vegetable water, stirring continuously. Return to the saucepan and cook until the sauce thickens. Add more cornflour if necessary. Season well. Remove from the heat and stir in the parsley.

Pour the sauce over the vegetables and mix well. Place the mixture in an ovenproof dish. Sprinkle the stuffing mix on top and bake in the oven for 15 minutes. Serve immediately.

MARINATED BROCCOLI AND PEPPER STIR-FRY WITH NOODLES

SERVES 4
PER SERVING 298 KCAL/7.1G FAT

225g (8oz) broccoli florets
2 medium red peppers
225g (8oz) beansprouts
225g (8oz) [dry weight] Chinese noodles

for the marinade
1 red onion, finely sliced
2 garlic cloves, crushed
1 × 2.5cm (1in) piece fresh ginger, finely chopped
3 tablespoons orange juice
1 tablespoon light soy sauce
1 teaspoon sesame seeds
1 teaspoon finely chopped chilli

Combine all the marinade ingredients in a large bowl.

Break the broccoli into bite-size pieces. Remove the seeds from the peppers and slice them into thin strips. Add the vegetables to the marinade and mix well. Leave for 10 minutes.

Meanwhile, place the noodles in a heatproof bowl and cover with boiling water. Allow them to stand for 5 minutes.

Preheat a non-stick wok. Remove the vegetables from the marinade, reserving the marinade. Stir-fry the marinated vegetables for 5–6 minutes until they start to soften. Add the beansprouts and cook for a further 2–3 minutes.

Drain the noodles and place in a saucepan. Add the reserved marinade and bring to the boil, combining well. Serve the vegetables and noodles immediately.

FENNEL AND TOMATO PASTA

SERVES 4
PER SERVING 292 KCAL/6.7G FAT

225g (8oz) [dry weight] pasta shapes
1 vegetable stock cube
1 medium onion, finely chopped
2 garlic cloves, crushed
50g (2oz) fresh fennel, finely sliced
2 teaspoons vegetable bouillon stock powder
600ml (1 pint) tomato passata
1 tablespoon chopped mixed herbs
4 teaspoons grated Parmesan cheese
salt and freshly ground black pepper

Cook the pasta in plenty of boiling water with the vegetable stock cube until tender.

Meanwhile, in a non-stick frying pan, dry-fry the onion until soft. Add the garlic and fennel and cook for a further 2–3 minutes.

Sprinkle with the stock powder and stir the passata and herbs into the pan. Cover, and simmer for 5 minutes.

Drain the pasta well and season with salt and black pepper. Pour into a warmed serving dish and spoon the sauce on top. Sprinkle with Parmesan cheese and serve with a mixed leaf salad.

CHILLI PASTA BAKE

SERVES 2
PER SERVING 500 KCAL/6.6G FAT

225g (8oz) [dry weight] pasta shapes
2 courgettes, diced
2 medium leeks, washed and diced
2 garlic cloves, crushed
1 red chilli, seeded and finely chopped
1 tablespoon chopped fresh oregano
1 tablespoon chopped fresh parsley
600ml (1 pint) tomato passata
2 tablespoons grated Parmesan
3 tablespoons low-fat natural yogurt
salt and freshly ground black pepper

Preheat the oven to 190C, 375F, Gas Mark 5.

Cook the pasta in boiling salted water until tender, then drain.

In a large non-stick saucepan dry-fry the courgette, leeks and garlic for 2–3 minutes. Add the chilli, herbs and passata. Stir in the cooked pasta and season to taste.

Transfer the mixture to an ovenproof dish and sprinkle with Parmesan. Bake in the oven for 30–35 minutes or until golden brown.

Just before serving, drizzle with the yogurt.

TAGLIATELLE WITH SUN-DRIED TOMATO AND CORIANDER PESTO

SERVES 2

PER SERVING 468 KCAL/6.2G FAT

65g (2½oz) sun-dried tomatoes (non-oil variety)
2 garlic cloves, crushed
1 tablespoon ground coriander
2 tablespoons chopped fresh coriander
300ml (½ pint) tomato passata
225g (8oz) [dry weight] tagliatelle
salt and freshly ground black pepper

Place all the ingredients except the pasta in a food processor and blend until smooth. Season to taste with salt and black pepper.

Cook the pasta in plenty of boiling salted water until tender, and drain.

Heat the tomato pesto in a saucepan for 2–3 minutes. Add the cooked pasta. Reheat and serve immediately.

Desserts and Cakes

HOT CHERRIES

SERVES 2

PER SERVING 129 KCAL/1.8G FAT

1 small tin (75g/3oz) black cherries in juice
50ml (2fl oz) cherry brandy
1 teaspoon slaked arrowroot
25g (1oz) Wall's 'Too Good To Be True' iced dessert

Drain the cherries, reserving the juice.

Heat the juice in a pan and add the cherry brandy. Mix the arrowroot with a little water and add sufficient to the pan to thicken the liquid to make a syrup. Stir in the cherries and heat through.

Place the iced dessert on 2 serving plates and spoon the cherry syrup over. Serve immediately.

APRICOT PLUM/DATE SOFTIE

SERVES 4

PER SERVING 73 KCAL/0.6G FAT

50g (2oz) fresh stoned dates
175g (6oz) fresh or dried (reconstituted) apricots
275g (10oz) thick low-fat natural yogurt
2 egg whites
2 tablespoons Canderel powder
2 plums or apricots, sliced
few sprigs of mint

Blend the dates and apricots with the yogurt in food processor or liquidiser until smooth.

Whisk the egg whites until they form stiff peaks then fold in the Canderel.

Carefully fold the date mixture into the egg white and spoon into 4 individual dishes. Leave to set.

Just before serving, decorate with the plum or apricot slices and the mint.

ORANGE AND GINGER PASHKA

SERVES 6

PER SERVING 113 KCAL/1G FAT

225g (8oz) low-fat cottage cheese
225g (8oz) quark
150ml (¼ pint) low-fat natural yogurt
2 pieces stem ginger in 2 tablespoons syrup
2 oranges
artificial sweetener to taste (optional)
small piece crystallised orange peel
extra piece stem ginger
small piece crystallised angelica leaf
2 ripe passion fruits

First prepare the mould. You will need either a small new flowerpot or a plastic yogurt or similar pot capable of holding about 500g (1¼lb). Punch several holes in the case (using a heated skewer is the easiest way to do this) and line with a piece of clean muslin. Set to one side until required.

Drain and discard any liquid from the cottage cheese. Using a wooden spoon, press or rub the cottage cheese and quark through a sieve into a bowl. Stir in the yogurt.

Chop the 2 pieces of stem ginger and reserve the syrup. Grate the rind from 1½ oranges. Cut the segments from 1 orange and reserve. Cut the other orange in half. Cut the segments from one half and chop coarsely. Squeeze the juice from the other half orange and reserve.

Stir the chopped ginger, grated orange rind, chopped flesh from the half orange and the reserved syrup from the stem ginger into the cheese mixture and mix well. Add a little artificial sweetener if you wish. Spoon the mixture into the prepared mould and smooth over the top. Wrap the edges of the muslin over the top. Place the mould on a pastry cutter in a bowl or shallow dish with a light weight on top (about 350–450g/12–16oz). Refrigerate overnight.

Prepare the decoration by cutting thin diamond or other shapes from the crystallised orange peel, the stem ginger and the crystallised angelica leaf. Cover with clingfilm until required.

The next day, turn the pashka out onto a serving dish. On the top of the pashka arrange a spiral of orange slices in the centre and a decorative edging of the crystallised fruit shapes. Just before serving, cut the passion fruits in half and, using a spoon, scoop out the centres. Mix with the reserved orange juice. Add a little sweetener to taste if you wish. Pour the juice around the edge of the pashka and serve.

RHUBARB AND ORANGE FOOL

SERVES 4
PER SERVING 101 KCAL/0.4G FAT

4 large oranges
400g (14oz) [trimmed weight]
rhubarb, cut into 2.5cm (1in) chunks
10g (¼oz) Canderel
115g (4oz) light fromage frais
orange segments and sprigs of fresh
mint to decorate (optional)

Thinly pare the rind from one of the oranges, in one long piece if possible, taking care not to remove any of the pith. Place the rind in a stainless steel or enamel saucepan, then remove all the pith from the orange.

Remove the rind and pith from the remaining oranges, then one at a time, remove the segments from all 4 oranges, holding the oranges over a bowl to catch the juice and cutting each segment free of the connecting white tissue with a sharp knife. Squeeze the remaining tissue to extract all the juice.

Add 4 tablespoons of the orange juice to the orange rind in the saucepan, then cover the bowl containing the orange segments and juice and chill until needed. Add the prepared rhubarb and the Canderel to the saucepan, cover the pan and cook over a moderate heat for 5–6 minutes or until the rhubarb is soft. Meanwhile, place a nylon or stainless steel sieve over a bowl.

When cooked, pour the rhubarb into the sieve to drain. Return the juice to the saucepan and boil gently until it is reduced to about 4 tablespoonfuls.

Place the drained rhubarb in a bowl and remove the orange rind, then add the reduced juice and stir well so that the rhubarb pieces break down into a thick purée. Cover and chill for 2–3 hours.

Thirty minutes before serving, drain the juice from the orange segments (this will not be needed, but can be drunk or used for another purpose).

Fold the fromage frais into the rhubarb. Spoon half of the orange segments into 4 serving glasses and top with half of the rhubarb fool, then repeat. Chill until ready to serve. Just before serving, decorate with orange segments and mint.

CRUNCHY TOPPED FRUIT FOOL

SERVES 4
PER SERVING 128 KCAL/5.6G FAT

25g (1oz) jumbo oats
2 teaspoons granulated sugar
225g (8oz) strawberries
300g (11oz) low-fat fromage frais
artificial sweetener to taste (optional)

Place a sheet of foil on the grill pan and spread the oats out on the foil. Sprinkle with the sugar. Lightly toast under the grill and allow to cool.

Reserve one strawberry for decorating. Hull and mash the remainder with a fork and stir into the fromage frais. Sweeten to taste with the sweetener if desired. Spoon into serving glasses and chill.

Cut the reserved strawberry into 4 small slices.

Just before serving, sprinkle the fruit fool with the toasted oat flakes and decorate each glass with a slice of strawberry.

TIRAMISU

SERVES 8
PER SERVING 76 KCAL/2.7G FAT

2 heaped teaspoons coffee granules or powder
2 teaspoons brandy
1 packet sponge fingers (approximately 12 fingers)
1 sachet Bird's Sugar-free Dream Topping
150ml (¼ pint) skimmed or semi-skimmed milk
350g (12oz) low-fat fromage frais
powdered drinking chocolate to decorate

Mix the coffee with the brandy and make up to 150m (¼ pint) with water. Reserve half the sponge fingers and dip the remainder in the brandied coffee. Arrange the brandied fingers on the base of a serving dish to form a layer.

Make up the Dream Topping with the milk and mix in the fromage frais. Spoon half the mixture over the sponge fingers in the dish. Dip the reserved sponge fingers in the remaining brandied coffee and place over the mixture in the dish. Top with the remaining fromage frais mix.

Just before serving, sprinkle a little powdered drinking chocolate on top.

TOFFEE YOGURT MERINGUES

MAKES 6 MERINGUES
PER MERINGUE 82 KCAL/0.3G FAT

1 × 150g (5oz) pot low-fat toffee yogurt
225g (8oz) low-fat fromage frais
6 meringue nests
a little cocoa powder or drinking chocolate
6 sprigs fresh mint to decorate

Swirl the toffee yogurt into the fromage frais. Do not worry if it is not fully mixed, as this gives an attractive swirly effect.

Just before serving, place 2 rounded tablespoonfuls of the yogurt and fromage frais mixture into each meringue nest and dust with a light sprinkling of cocoa powder or drinking chocolate. Decorate each with a sprig of mint.

If you are not serving all the meringue nests at once, you can keep the yogurt and fromage frais mixture in the refrigerator for up to 4 days and then fill the nests when required.

BAKED BANANAS WITH RASPBERRIES

SERVES 2
PER SERVING 118 KCAL/0.5G FAT

115g (4oz) fresh or frozen raspberries
2 bananas
4 tablespoons orange juice

If using frozen raspberries, allow them to thaw.

Preheat the oven to 180C, 350F, Gas Mark 4. Peel the bananas and cut in half lengthways. Place each banana on a sheet of foil that is large enough to enclose it during cooking. Divide the raspberries between the 2 parcels and add 2 tablespoons of orange juice to each parcel. Fold up to enclose the fruit.

Place on a baking sheet and bake in the oven for 15 minutes. Remove from the oven and serve each one in its foil parcel.

BAKED EGG CUSTARD

SERVES 2
PER SERVING 109 KCAL/5.6G FAT

300ml (½ pint) skimmed milk
2 egg yolks
sugar or sweetener to taste
a little nutmeg (optional)

Preheat the oven to 160C, 325F, Gas Mark 2. Place the milk in a pan and heat until it 'steams'.

Lightly beat the egg yolks in a bowl until smooth.

Pour the hot milk onto the eggs and mix well. Sweeten to taste with sugar or sweetener. Strain into a small pie dish and sprinkle a little nutmeg over (if using).

Half-fill a small roasting tin with water. Place the pie dish in the roasting tin and place in the oven. Bake for about 1 hour until the custard is set and firm to touch.

BAKED STUFFED APPLE

SERVES 1
PER SERVING 100 KCAL/0.3G FAT

1 large cooking apple
25g (1oz) dried fruit
1 teaspoon honey

Preheat the oven to 200C, 400F, Gas Mark 6. Remove the core from the apple but leave the apple intact. Score with a sharp knife around the 'waist' of the apple, cutting through only the skin.

Mix together the dried fruit and the honey and pile into the centre of the apple. Place in an ovenproof dish and bake in the oven for about 30 minutes.

BAKED BANANA

SERVES 1
PER SERVING 103 KCAL/0.2G FAT

1 banana
pinch of brown sugar
1 tablespoon raisins
pinch of cinnamon

Preheat the oven to 180C, 350F, Gas Mark 4. Peel and slice the banana and place in a shallow ovenproof dish. Sprinkle with the brown sugar, raisins and cinnamon. Pour 4 tablespoons water over the banana and bake in the oven for 30 minutes.

GINGER MARMALADE CAKE

SERVES 10
PER SERVING 204 KCAL/1G FAT

This cake tends to eat better 2–3 days after making. Store in an airtight container or wrap well in grease-proof paper.

225g (8oz) mixed dried fruit
300ml (½ pint) cold tea
225g (8oz) self-raising flour
115g (4oz) caster sugar
1 egg, beaten
3 tablespoons ginger marmalade
1 tablespoon molasses
1 teaspoon ground ginger

Soak the mixed fruit in the tea overnight until the fruit swells.

Preheat the oven to 180C, 350F, Gas Mark 4. Line a 675g (1½lb) loaf tin with greaseproof paper, or use a non-stick tin.

In a bowl, combine the flour, sugar, egg and marmalade, then add the molasses and ground ginger. Mix well and place in the loaf tin. Bake in the oven for 1 hour.

Leave to cool before slicing.

PRUNE AND ALMOND CAKE

SERVES 8
PER SERVING 206 KCAL/2.6G FAT

225g (8oz) ready-to-eat prunes
175g (6oz) plain flour
2 teaspoons baking powder
175g (6oz) caster sugar
3 eggs
2 teaspoons mixed spice
1 teaspoon almond essence
icing sugar to serve

Soak the prunes in a mug of hot black tea overnight.

Preheat the oven to 180C, 350F, Gas Mark 4. Line a 900g (2lb) loaf tin with greaseproof paper.

Drain the soaked prunes and purée half of them in a food processor or liquidiser. Mix the prune purée with the flour, baking powder, sugar, eggs and spice in a large bowl.

Chop the remaining prunes and fold the chopped prunes and almond essence into the mixture in the bowl.

Pour the mixture into the loaf tin and bake in the oven for 35–40 minutes.

Dust with icing sugar before serving.

CARROT AND MANGO CAKE

SERVES 10
PER SERVING 207 KCAL/1.1G FAT

225g (8oz) plain flour
3 heaped teaspoons baking powder
175g (6oz) dark brown soft sugar
1 teaspoon ground ginger
1 teaspoon ground coriander
1 teaspoon mixed spice
115g (4oz) sultanas
115g (4oz) fresh mangoes, diced
450g (1lb) carrots, grated
1 egg, beaten
250ml (8fl oz) skimmed or semi-skimmed milk

for the topping
115g (4oz) quark
zest of 1 orange
115g (4oz) icing sugar
a few poppy seeds

Preheat the oven to 180C, 350F, Gas Mark 4. Line a 450g (1lb) round cake tin with greaseproof paper or baking parchment, or use a non-stick tin.

In a bowl, mix together the flour, baking powder, sugar, ground ginger, coriander, spice, sultanas and diced mangoes. Add the grated carrots and stir well.

Mix the beaten egg with the milk. Stir into the mixture and mix well. Pour the mixture into the prepared tin and bake in the oven for 50–55 minutes. To test if the cake is cook, insert a skewer into the cake. The skewer should come out clean.

Leave to cool before serving. Just before serving, make the topping by mixing together the quark, orange zest and icing sugar until smooth. Spread over the top of the cake. Sprinkle with poppy seeds.

APPLE GATEAU

SERVES 8
PER SERVING 192 KCAL/3.3G FAT

75g (3oz) plain flour
3 eggs
125g (4 1/2oz) caster sugar
pinch of salt
1 teaspoon icing sugar
for the filling
450g (1lb) eating apples
zest and juice of 1 lemon
1 tablespoon apricot jam
artificial sweetener to taste (optional)

Preheat the oven to 190C, 375F, Gas Mark 5. Very lightly grease an 20cm (8in) cake tin. Dust with a little caster sugar then with a little flour. Shake out the excess.

Sift the flour. Place the eggs and caster sugar in a mixing bowl and whisk with an electric whisk or mixer for 5 minutes at top speed until thick and mousse-like. Fold in the sifted flour and salt. Pour the mixture into the prepared tin. Bake in the centre of the oven for 25 minutes or until the cake is golden brown and has shrunk from the edges of the tin a little. Run a blunt knife around the inside of the tin and turn out the cake onto a wire rack to cool.

To make the filling, peel and slice the apples and place the apple slices in a saucepan. Add the lemon zest and juice and the jam. Heat slowly. Add artificial sweetener to taste if required. Cover and cook until the apples are just tender. Allow to cool.

When the cake is cool, slice it across with a large knife to make 2 layers. Spread the bottom half with the cooled apple filling and cover with the top half of the cake. Sprinkle the cake with icing sugar.

SPICY FRUIT AND APPLE CAKE

SERVES 10
PER SERVING 205 KCAL/1G FAT

350g (12oz) dried mixed fruit
150ml (¼ pint) hot black tea
175g (6oz) soft brown sugar
115g (4oz) cooking apples, diced
350g (12oz) self-raising flour
1 egg, beaten
2 teaspoons mixed spice
1 teaspoon ground cinnamon

Soak the dried fruit in the hot tea overnight.

Preheat the oven to 170C, 325F, Gas Mark 3. Line a 900g (2lb) loaf tin or round cake tin with greaseproof paper.

Place the soaked fruit in a bowl and add the remaining ingredients. Combine well. Transfer the mixture to the prepared loaf or cake tin and bake in the oven for 2 hours.

When cooked, leave the cake to cool in the tin.

BRAN LOAF

SERVES 6
PER SERVING 193 KCAL/0.5G FAT

1 cup branflakes or All-Bran
1 cup sultanas
1 cup skimmed milk
½ cup brown sugar
pinch of mixed spice (optional)
1 cup wholemeal self-raising flour

Place all the ingredients except the flour in a bowl and leave for 1 hour.

Preheat the oven to 170C, 325F, Gas Mark 3. Lightly grease a 450g (1lb) loaf tin and line the base with greaseproof paper.

Add the flour to the bran mixture in the bowl and stir well. Place in the prepared loaf tin and bake in the oven for 1 hour 10 minutes.

Remove from the oven, turn out onto a wire rack and leave to cool.

VANILLA SWISS ROLL WITH LEMON CURD

SERVES 6

PER SERVING 197 KCAL/2.3G FAT

2 eggs
75g (3oz) self-raising flour
75g (3oz) sugar
fine zest of 1 lemon
1 teaspoon vanilla essence
for the lemon curd
fine zest and juice of 4 lemons
450ml ($^3/_4$ pint) skimmed milk
2 tablespoons custard powder
$1^1/_2$ tablespoons caster sugar

Preheat the oven to 180C, 350F, Gas Mark 4. Line a non-stick swiss roll tin with parchment paper.

Whisk the eggs in a bowl for several minutes until thick and creamy and pale in consistency. Sift the flour and, using a metal spoon, carefully fold the flour and sugar into the eggs, then fold in the lemon zest and the vanilla. Pour quickly into the prepared swiss roll tin. Bake in the oven for 25–30 minutes until golden brown and firm to the touch.

When cooked, turn the sponge out onto sugared greaseproof paper and roll up with the paper. Leave to cool with paper still wrapped around the roll.

To make the lemon curd, place the lemon zest and juice in a measuring jug and make up to 600ml (1 pint) with skimmed milk. Mix the custard powder and sugar with a little of the lemon mixture into a paste.

Place the remainder of the lemon mixture in a saucepan and bring to the boil. Pour onto the custard powder, mix well and return to the pan. Bring back to the boil, whisking continuously until the curd thickens. Allow to cool.

When the lemon curd is completely cool, unroll the sponge, remove the parchment paper, and spread the lemon curd mixture onto the sponge and roll up again.

Dressings

BALSAMIC DRESSING

MAKES 180ML (6½FL OZ)
PER TABLESPOON 12 KCAL/0.2G FAT

150ml (¼ pint) apple juice
2 tablespoons balsamic vinegar
1 tablespoon Dijon mustard
pinch of sugar
salt and freshly ground black pepper

Combine all ingredients in a small bowl and whisk until smooth. Place in a sealed jar or bottle and use as required. Use within 5 days.

FAT-FREE MAYONNAISE

MAKES 220ML (7¹/₂FL OZ))
PER TABLESPOON 9 KCAL/0.02G FAT

175g (6oz) virtually fat free fromage-frais
2 tablespoons cider vinegar
1 tablespoon lemon juice
¹/₄ teaspoon ground turmeric
2 teaspoons sugar
salt and freshly ground black pepper

Combine all the ingredients together in a small bowl and whisk until smooth. Place in a sealed container, store in the refrigerator and use within 3 days.

GARLIC AND YOGURT DRESSING

SERVES 4
PER SERVING 20 KCAL/0.3G FAT

1 garlic clove, crushed
150g (5oz) low-fat natural yogurt
1 tablespoon white wine vinegar
1 teaspoon reduced-oil salad dressing
salt and freshly ground black pepper to taste

Mix all the ingredients together in a container, seal, and shake well. Taste and add more salt or sugar as desired.

HONEY AND ORANGE DRESSING

MAKES 150ML (¼ PINT)
PER TABLESPOON 11 KCAL/0.02G FAT

6 tablespoons orange juice
4 teaspoons thin honey
1 tablespoon white wine vinegar
½ teaspoon Dijon wholegrain mustard
1 teaspoon grated orange rind
2 teaspoons chopped fresh chives and
parsley, mixed
salt and freshly ground black pepper to taste.

Place the orange juice, honey and vinegar in a pan. Add
the Dijon mustard and orange rind. Bring to the boil,
then allow to cool.

When cool, add the chopped chives and parsley and
season to taste with salt and black pepper. Place in a
bottle or jar, seal the top and place in the refrigerator.
Use within 7 days.

MARIE ROSE DRESSING

SERVES 2
PER SERVING 73 KCAL/1G FAT

2 tablespoons tomato ketchup
1 tablespoon reduced-oil salad dressing
4 tablespoons low-fat natural yogurt
dash of Tabasco sauce
salt and freshly ground black pepper to taste

Mix all the ingredients together and store in a sealed jar in the refrigerator. Use within 2 days.

OIL-FREE VINAIGRETTE

MAKES 200ML (7FL OZ)
PER TABLESPOON 9 KCAL/0.1G FAT

150ml ($\frac{1}{4}$ pint) white wine vinegar or cider vinegar
50ml (2fl oz) lemon juice
3–4 teaspoons caster sugar
$1\frac{1}{2}$ teaspoons French mustard
chopped fresh herbs, e.g. marjoram, basil
or parsley (optional)
1 garlic clove, crushed (optional)
$\frac{1}{2}$ teaspoon salt
$\frac{1}{2}$ teaspoon freshly ground black pepper

Mix all the ingredients together and pour into a screw top jar or other container with a tight-fitting lid. Shake well. Taste and add more salt, pepper or sugar if you wish. Store in the refrigerator and shake well before using.

Index

Weekly Exercise Planner

Indicate which times you are going to set aside to do your Healthy Heart Programme and your Muscle Training Programme. Aim to do the Healthy Heart Programme at least three times a week and the Muscle Training Programme at least twice a week.

	MONDAY	TUESDAY	WEDNESDAY	THURSDAY	FRIDAY	SATURDAY	SUNDAY
MORNING SESSION Healthy Heart Programme 30 mins	☐	☐	☐	☐	☐	☐	☐
LUNCHTIME SESSION Healthy Heart Programme 30 mins	☐	☐	☐	☐	☐	☐	☐
Muscle Training Session 15 mins	☐	☐	☐	☐	☐	☐	☐
AFTERNOON SESSION Healthy Heart Programme 30 mins	☐	☐	☐	☐	☐	☐	☐
EVENING SESSION Muscle Training Session 15 mins	☐	☐	☐	☐	☐	☐	☐

THE RED WINE DIET

	WEIGHT NOW	POUNDS LOST	TOTAL LOSS TO DATE
START DAY Date:			
WEEK 1 Date:			
WEEK 2 Date:			
WEEK 3 Date:			
WEEK 4 Date:			
WEEK 5 Date:			
WEEK 6 Date:			
WEEK 7 Date:			
WEEK 8 Date:			
WEEK 9 Date:			
WEEK 10 Date:			
WEEK 11 Date:			
WEEK 12 Date:			
TOTAL LOST			

WEIGHT AND INCH LOSS RECORD

WAIST MEASUREMENT	INCHES / CM LOST TO DATE	NOTES

Rosemary Conley

DIET & FITNESS CLUBS

DIET AND FITNESS CLASSES THAT COMBINE A HEALTHY LOW-FAT DIET WITH SAFE AND EFFECTIVE EXERCISE SUITABLE FOR EVERYONE

Rosemary Conley Clubs offer you the chance to shape up, slim down and transform your body as you never thought possible!

Follow Rosemary Conley's diet in the company of others – just like you – and benefit from weekly exercise, encouragement, advice and support. At every Rosemary Conley Club class, members weigh in and work out under the supervision of a qualified instructor. The diet is easy to follow and proven to work, while the exercise session can be adapted to cater for everyone, no matter what their age, weight, or fitness level.

Whether you have a lot or just a little weight to lose, our specially trained instructors will ensure you are made very welcome, and you will receive all the help and encouragement you need. It's an enjoyable and sociable way to shed your excess weight, lose inches and achieve a fitter and healthier lifestyle.

TOGETHER WE CAN DO IT!

For details of classes in your area, ring

01509 620222

Caltrac™

At last – a gadget that tells you how many calories you are burning as you burn them!

Space-age technology applied to energy expenditure, Caltrac gives you the motivation to do more activity to help you lose more weight, more quickly.

Caltrac measures the calories you BURN. This has been the *missing part* of the weight-control equation. You just enter your individual details – height, weight, age and sex – and Caltrac does the rest. It calculates your basal metabolic rate and clocks up the calories as you burn them. It enables you to learn how you can burn more calories each day through activity. The more energetic you are, the more your total goes up. It makes you think twice before eating something extra, as well as motivating you to do more exercise.

Caltrac is like having a personal trainer. It is revolutionary, it's clever and it's a great help when you are trying to lose weight. It's tough and has a practically unbreakable ABS plastic case, easy five button controls and a handy waist-clip.

The recommended retail price is £70. Here's your chance to order it at the very special price of just £45 (including p&p). That's a saving of £25.

Caltrac has been used by many undergraduates and in post-graduate courses in exercise science.

To order your Caltrac monitor, just send your order form and payment to:
Rosemary Conley Enterprises,
Quorn House,
Meeting Street,
Quorn,
Leicestershire LE12 8EX

or use the credit card hotline number below.

☎ **Credit Card Hotline 01509 620444** (Mon–Fri 9–5pm)

Please complete in BLOCK CAPITALS and return to:
Rosemary Conley's Office, Rosemary Conley Enterprises, Quorn House, Meeting
Street, Quorn, Leicestershire, LE12 8EX.

Please send me:	Quantity	Unit price	Total £
Caltrac		£45.00	

PLEASE INDICATE QUANTITY AND TOTAL

PLEASE USE BLOCK CAPITALS

Mr/Mrs/Miss/Ms (Initials) _____ Surname _____

Address _____

_____

_____

Postcode _____

Daytime Tel. No. (in case of query) _____

I enclose a crossed cheque/postal order made payable to Rosemary Conley

Enclose for £ _____ OR please debit my Switch/Mastercard/Visa/Delta

(delete as appropriate) with the sum of £ _____

Card No

☐☐☐☐☐ ☐☐☐☐☐ ☐☐☐☐☐ ☐☐☐☐☐

Issue No. (Switch only) _____

Valid from _____ expires _____ Signature _____

Allow 28 days from receipt of order for delivery.
Offer applies to UK applicants (including Northern Ireland and Channel Islands) only.